SpringerBriefs in Philosophy

For further volumes:
http://www.springer.com/series/10082

Jennifer Bullington

The Expression of the Psychosomatic Body from a Phenomenological Perspective

Springer

Jennifer Bullington
Ersta Sköndal University College
Stockholm
Sweden

ISSN 2211-4548 ISSN 2211-4556 (electronic)
ISBN 978-94-007-6497-2 ISBN 978-94-007-6498-9 (eBook)
DOI 10.1007/978-94-007-6498-9
Springer Dordrecht Heidelberg New York London

Library of Congress Control Number: 2013933017

Printed on acid-free paper

Springer is part of Springer Science+Business Media (www.springer.com)

Contents

Introduction

The patient who presents somatic symptoms with no clearly discernible lesion or dysfunction presents a problem to the traditional health care system. These symptoms are medically unexplainable (so-called "MUS" = medically unexplained symptoms) and thus constitute an anomaly for the materialistic understanding of health problems that underlies the practice of modern medicine. The history of Western medicine is the story of how the body gradually revealed its internal mysteries, after human dissection was approved, (formally permitted in 1565 at London's Royal College of Physicians), resulting in the conceptualization of disease and ill health in terms of identifiable abnormalities in the body. The discovery of viruses and bacteria further solidified the explanatory power of material "stuff" in the body as pathogenic, while the coming of modern technologies allowed for an even further level of material discernment by augmenting the eye of the doctor through sophisticated machinery and laboratory tests. These advances have made possible the cure and prevention of many diseases and are very useful for those conditions that can be properly understood in material terms. However, this traditional biomedical model is not appropriate for understanding a number of health issues that we call "psychosomatic" and for this reason, biomedical theory and practice must be complemented in order to adequately understand and treat the psychosomatic anomaly. This book is an attempt to establish a complementary understanding of health and illness in terms of a non-reductionist model allowing for the psychosomatic expression of the lived body. The term "lived body" comes from the philosophy of Maurice Merleau-Ponty, and it is his work which will be the theoretical inspiration for the alternative understanding of psychosomatics worked out in these chapters.

Chapter 1
The Psychosomatic Problematic

The philosophical so-called "mind–body problem" lies at the core of the psychosomatic problematic. The relationship between the mental and the material, meaning and matter, has been a philosophical issue as long as man has reflected on his own being. However, the relationship between the mind and the body in terms of ill health became a problem first when ill health was conceptualized in terms of material lesions and dysfunction in the somatic body. In Ancient Greece and China, for example, health and illness were understood in holistic terms, where balanced relations with others and with nature were just as important for health as eating right and exercising. But when the cause of ill health is reduced to one part of the whole (the material), our view of health and illness becomes limited to a reductionist framework. Within this framework, it is not hard to understand how a broken bone causes pain, or how glucose levels affect a diabetic. But it is no longer comprehensible to say how a bad marriage "causes" bad health. Because of the focus on the somatic (materiality of the body) as the source of ill health, we have a clinical problem as well. Not only is medical practice primarily concerned with the material body, the patient with psychosomatic problems has also formed his/her understanding of health problems in somatic terms. Because of this somatic focus, psychosocial problems are not understood as such, but rather present themselves to the person with the "psychosomatic solution" and to the health care professional solely in terms of somatic complaints, which most often do not have any discernible material causes. In such a case, the patient has fixated on a level of expression (the body symptom) which is inadequate to the task of mediating the psychosocial problem, and the health care professional has nothing in his/her repertoire that will have any effect on the somatic symptom, since the health problem has its source in the life of the patient, not in the material of the body. As long as the challenge in the life of the patient remains unattended to, the symptoms will remain. This is, in short, the psychosomatic problematic. The way in which something belonging to "meaning" (the way in which people understand and live their lives) gets translated into something somatic/material is what Freud called

J. Bullington, *The Expression of the Psychosomatic Body from a Phenomenological Perspective*, SpringerBriefs in Philosophy,
DOI: 10.1007/978-94-007-6498-9_1,

"the mysterious leap to the somatic".[1] This leap remains mysterious and is the central problem to be explained in all traditional psychosomatic theory. However, the "leap" is unnecessary if we abstain from splitting up man into an objective somatic material body and an immaterial, subjective realm of meaning constitution. This will become clear in connection with the work of Merleau-Ponty presented in the following chapters.

The ultimate failure of psychosomatic theory lies in the dualistic[2] conceptualization of man as being made up of two distinct realms that have seemingly mutually exclusive characteristics. That which is "mind" is subjective, private, non-spatial, qualitative, intentional, privileged access (known only to me). Mind has to do with feelings, attitudes, values, self—awareness, intentions and so on. The material (the body) is characterized as the opposite of the mental, i.e. as that which is objective, public, spatial, quantitative (measurable) and mechanical. In this way, the inside (mind) and the outside (body) constitute two essentially different orders of reality, united in one being. Throughout history man has grappled with how this union can be understood. In this context, however, suffice to say that as long as one has a conception of the body as "meaningless" material and the mind as the opposite of the body, psychosomatic conditions will remain inexplicable.

The theoretical attempt to understand the psychosomatic relation in modern times can be traced back to three traditional psychosomatic traditions (psychodynamic, psychosomatic medicine, stress theory) with roots in the beginning of the 1900s. These three orientations had overlapping boundaries in the early phase of development from the 1930s, but later on these traditions developed into distinct approaches with different ontological and etiological positions regarding psychosomatics. The psychodynamic tradition, with the concept of conversion hysteria first formulated by Freud, had a connection to the early writings of psychosomatic medicine, since Franz Alexander, one of the founding fathers of psychosomatic medicine, was also a psychoanalyst, exerting a strong influence on the early work in this tradition. However, after the failure of Alexander's "specificity hypothesis" (the attempt to correlate specific psychological conflicts with specific psychosomatic diseases) theoreticians within psychosomatic medicine gradually abandoned psychoanalytic theory and concerned themselves with trying to establish correlations between biological, psychological and social factors related to health and

---

[1] The term was first used by Freudin "The Rat Man" paper from 1909. See also "[...] the leap from a mental process to a somatic innervations- hysterical conversion—which can never be fully comprehensible to us" Freud (1909), p. 157.

[2] The term dualism comes from the Latin *dualis* which means two-fold. Dualism states that the world is made up of two kinds of essences, that which is spirit or mind (immaterial) and that which is material. The opposite of dualism is monism, which maintains that there is only one basic "stuff" in the universe. A monistic position on the mind–body problem would be that minds and brains are made up of the same substance. Although dualists are in agreement about the dual nature of reality, there are controversies among them regarding the nature of the relationship between the material and the immaterial and their interdependence.

illness. Stress researchers were primarily interested in the physiology of stress. The earliest work in stress research performed by Walter Canon and Hans Selye in the 1930s concerned experimental work on rats, however this tradition eventually evolved into human-focused research thanks to the psychological work of James Mason (1975) in the 1970s and the appraisal theory of stress proposed by Richard Lazarus and Susan Folkman (1984) in the 1980s. I wrote above that these traditional theories have all failed to give a comprehensible account of the psychosomatic, and in order to justify that claim I will very briefly give an account of the theoretical dead-ends in these traditions before returning to the psychosomatic problematic facing health care today.

Summary of Traditional Psychosomatic Theories

The psychodynamic theory of psychosomatics has remained basically unchanged since the writings of Freud. Modern proponents, such as Joyce McDougal (1985, 1989) still embrace the conversion hypothesis ("conversion hysteria" was the term for what we today call "psychosomatic"), a process whereby something from the mind is said to be converted into the body (a bodily symptom). The hypothesis is that an unconscious, repressed wish or fantasy has a "charge" or energy surrounding it, and this energy builds up in the unconscious since the person is unable to discharge[3] it via "normal" paths such as thoughts, feelings and actions, as the "mental" representation (meaning component) is unconscious. The idea is that psychical energy surrounding forbidden ideas and wishes, if it becomes too strong, will eventually get discharged into the body, giving rise to the psychosomatic bodily symptoms. In Freud's first model of conversion, this "leakage" into the body was thought to be due a so-called "somatic compliance" consisting of a congenital weakness or organic predisposition, meaning that the symptom will appear at the body's weakest link. However, later on he noticed that the symptom seemed to have symbolic meaning which could be interpreted. The etiology of this conversion process, in order to be comprehensible, is dependent on the so-called economical model of the psyche, where the psyche is conceptualized as a sort of enclosed hydraulic system. In this system, built up pressure must be discharged

[3] Freud called this discharge "abreaction" which entails the idea that psychical energy must be dissipated in order to maintain psychical equilibrium. Normal abreaction occurs, for example, after trauma and/or inner conflict, if one can react with emotions or actions, or if one manages to resolve inner psychical conflict through reflection or modification of values. When these options are not available, the psychical energy surrounding repressed unconscious ideas or memories becomes pathogenic, causing neuroses, or in the case of conversion hysteria, leads to the formation of somatic symptoms.

(through thoughts, feelings or actions) in order to maintain psychological health.[4] Freud intended to address the nature of this conversion process in his *Preliminaries to a Metapsychology,* a book that was to contain twelve papers addressing various theoretical problems which had arisen during the first decades of psychoanalytic practice. Five of the twelve papers were actually written, published in 1915 as the *Papers on Metapsychology,* but the remaining seven were never written or destroyed. Conversion hysteria was to be the subject of one of these lost or abandoned papers. Apparently, the mystery was too hard to solve within the framework of Freud's metapsychology, so he left it to others.[5]

The authors within the psychodynamic tradition who deal with mind–body issues fall in line with a form of "identity-theory" of the mind/brain problematic, where psychical processes are said to exist, in their own right, demanding their own methods and forms of understanding, yet at the same time it is assumed that the psychical is just "another side" of neurophysiological processes. The nature of the relationship between the psychical and the neurophysiological was a problem that neither Freud nor any of his disciples could solve.[6] Modern neuropsychoanalysis, through the work of Solms (Solms 1997; Solms and Turnbull 2002) and others, has proposed a materialistic theory of the relationship between mind and brain without addressing materialisms reductionistic perspective. The failure to adequately define "the mental/psychical" within a materialistic framework leads to a confusion in the theory, where the mind and the brain are often used interchangeably (as if they were the same), or alternatively, the term "brain" is used when what is actually described is a psychical act, having nothing to do with the brain as a material organ. The brain in this theory often acts as little "person" (a homunculus) and is ascribed characteristics that belong to persons, not brains. The philosophical problems associated with materialism will be further explicated in connection to the discussion of psychosomatic medicine.

According to psychodynamic theory, that which is efficacious in the formation of psychosomatic symptoms is ultimately those physiological processes associated with the psychical level of signification (meaning), for example, the energy surrounding forbidden repressed thought and feelings. The only thing that can "cause" psychosomatic symptoms is either psychical energy (*cathexis* surrounding repressed ideas, wishes and fantasies) or repressed emotions, according to this theory. Emotions are conceivable causes of psychosomatic symptoms because they

[4] It is unclear whether or not we have a different form of energy involved in the symptom formation. If the energy is the same, "conversion" is a misleading term, as it suggests a transformation from one kind of energy into another. If all that has happened is that this energy has changed its route, it would be more proper to speak of "diversion".

[5] See "Editors introduction" to *Papers on Metapsychology* (1950) pp. 105–107 on the missing metapsychological papers.

[6] Felix Deutsch (1959) devoted an entire book to "the riddle of the mind–body correlations" as he called it, written in celebration of the centenary of Freud 's birth, consisting of a number of psychoanalysts discussing in workshop form what Freud could have meant by the "mysterious leap" and how they themselves attempted to understand the issue.

are good examples of "frontier concepts"[7] which have both physiological and psychological components. The idea of using emotions as a bridge between mind and body is a strategy which almost all traditional theories have had to use in order to try and find a comprehensible link between meaning (psychosocial realm) and the physical body. That which is specific to the psychodynamic theory of psychosomatic pathology is the hypothesis of unconscious conflicts and their accompanying psychical energy (*cathexis*). Without the unconscious, there is no psycho*dynamic* theory (i.e. the conflicts between the Id, the Ego and the Superego) and without the economical pillar of the Metapsychology there is no conceivable way to understand the formation of psychosomatic symptoms. As we shall see later on, there are sound intuitions within this theoretical tradition that are useful to psychosomatics, such as the notion of balance (however not in terms of hydraulic "abreaction"), the symbolic significance of the symptom (the speaking body), and the curative role of verbalization. But these insights will have to be reformulated within another framework in order to be comprehensible.

The basic problem with the psychodynamic theory of conversion hysteria, even if one accepts the notion of the unconscious and the economic theory of discharge, is the description of symptom formation from a dualistic perspective. In the Freudian system, man is conceptualized as being at the mercy of "forces" or "energies" in need of "abreaction" (energy discharge needed in order to sustain psychical equilibrium) and as such, passive and "thing-like" as well as the active, wishing creature, motivated by desires. The mind–body problem arises then in yet another form, as the relationship between forces and meaning needs explication. Ricoeur (1970) has pointed out that there is something paradoxical about the Freudian dual characterization of man, since one can neither interpret forces nor quantify desire (qua desire). One may resolve the paradox by simply taking sides for one of the other aspect (explanation in terms of energy or understanding in terms of meaning), but Freud wanted to have both. To sum up, the development of the psychodynamic theory of psychosomatics has been hindered by the dualistic characterization of man and its adherence to the incomprehensible conversion premise. Freud himself formulated the problem clearly:

> We know two kinds of things about what we call our psyche (or mental life); firstly, its bodily organ and scene of action, the brain (or nervous system) and, on the other hand, our acts of consciousness, which are immediate data and cannot be further explained by any sort of description. Everything that lies between is unknown to us, and the data do not include any direct relation between these two terminal points of our knowledge. If it existed, it would at the most afford an exact localization of the processes of consciousness and would give us no help towards understanding them (1938/1940, p. 144).

[7] The notion of a frontier concept comes from Freud's discussion of the nature of the instinctual drive as being "a concept on the frontier between the somatic and the mental" (Freud 1915 SE Vol. XIV, pp. 121–122). See also Editor's Introduction to SE Vol. XIV pp. 111 ff on the "frontier concept" of the instinct and the ambiguity of its ontological status.

Psychosomatic medicine,[8] as the branch of Western medicine specifically concerned with mind–body relations has a short history, usually dated from the publication in 1935 of Flanders Dunbar's (1935) and the first appearance in 1939 of the *Journal of Psychosomatic Medicine*. Dunbar's book was an attempt to collect and synthesize all available literature up to that time (2251 articles) on the relationship between somatic functioning and the emotions. The intention of the *Journal of Psychosomatic Medicine* was to delineate this new psychosomatic field of study and set up guidelines for further medical research. The "Introductory Statement" in the first issue of the journal (Alexander 1939), often quoted and referred to, can be seen as a kind of credo, which to this day is more or less regarded as the official position of psychosomatic medicine. The Statement defines the role of psychosomatic medicine as follows: "Its object is to study in their interrelation the psychological and physiological aspects of all normal and abnormal bodily functions and thus to integrate somatic therapy and psychotherapy." (*Journal of Psychosomatic Medicine* 1:3.)

The field of psychosomatic medicine was dominated by psychoanalytic theory from the 1930s until the mid-1950s. This orientation led to an emphasis placed upon the importance of psychological factors on somatic functioning. As mentioned earlier, the psychoanalyst Franz Alexander had a strong influence on the development of psychosomatic theory within psychosomatic medicine in the early phase. But when his attempt to correlate specific unconscious conflicts with specific diseases and illnesses proved to be unfruitful, a shift was made in the 1950s from the psychodynamic interest in intra-psychic conflicts, motivations and defenses to a psycho-physiological approach, focusing on the so-called "mediating mechanisms" between symbolic "stimuli" and their physiological response. The turn from psychoanalytic theory towards natural scientific language and ideals is clear in the literature from the 1970s onward. The psycho-physiological approach can be said to be a modern version of the well-known theme of the negative impact of the passions on the body.[9] In modern thinking, strong emotions alone are not considered sufficient causes of disease, but they are one of the variables (an extremely important one) which may intervene between man and his environment in a detrimental way.

A current version of the theme of detrimental effects of emotions in psychosomatic medicine can be seen in Denollet's (2005) construct "type D personality" where the D stands for "distressed". Persons with this personality type are said to be inclined towards negative emotions, such as worry, irritability and gloom as well as exhibiting social inhibition. They lack the ability to share their distress with

---

[8] The texts used for this analysis are those within the tradition that attempt to formulate a theoretical understanding of psychosomatics, not the empirical studies. The texts are the so-called classical ones, as well as those written by prominent writers in the field.

[9] The idea that the passions have a detrimental impact on health is referred to in the medical textbooks of the seventeenth and eighteenth centuries. See Bynum and Porter (1993), Magretts (1954). In traditional Chinese medicine, strong emotions are generally to be avoided in order to maintain health.

others due to fear of rejection, which leads to suppressed emotions and further social isolation. Research has shown a correlation of this type of personality with heart problems, where Type D personalities have been found in up to 53 % of cardiac patients (Pedersen and Denollet 2006). These persons also have a tendency of somatic complains as children (Jellesma 2008). This is reminiscent of Alexander's idea that suppressed emotions are the cause of many forms of ill health that we call "psychosomatic".

To study mind and body in their interrelation is the credo of psychosomatic medicine. Disease processes, and indeed all health disorders, are considered to be the product of complex interactions between factors found in various interdependent systems. These systems (bio-physiological, psychological, social and cultural) are said to interact with each other via feedback loops, mutually intervening upon each other. Mechanisms of interaction between man and his world are found on all levels, from the cellular up to the socio-cultural. The etiology of disease is considered multi-factorial, that is to say, rarely is one mechanism or variable entirely responsible for the outbreak of disease. Complex patterns of interactions emerge. We find that subjective factors are important, specifically the traits and personality of the patient, his or her coping ability at the time of the onset of the disease, the cognitive and behavior patterns which may contribute to the inability to cope. The way in which intervening mechanisms intervene, however, remains unclear. Terms such as "influence", "activate", "induce", "result in" and "cause" are found in the literature, although the only comprehensible explication of interaction can be seen in the cases when specific factors somehow initiate and maintain (or hinder the reduction of) prolonged physiological arousal. The detrimental effect of sustained arousal is a recurrent etiological theme in the literature. Emotions are seen as a "link" between subjective meaning constitution and the physiology of the body, similar to the way in which psychoanalysts found emotions to be a convenient explanatory factor in psychosomatic pathology (although for different reasons). However, for the theory to work, emotions must be strong emotions, which are suppressed during a long period of time. The more subtle emotions (jealousy, envy, irritation, rivalry) have no efficacious explanatory value, since they do not "wear and tear" on the organism in the same way as strong emotions.

Theoreticians in psychosomatic medicine want to demonstrate causal relationships through verified hypotheses, true to the scientific ideals of the natural sciences. However, there are several inherent conflicts in the discipline of psychosomatic medicine that need to be brought out. The first conflict is between their "holistic approach[10] to man and the dualistic "interrelations" project.[11]

[10] The term "holistic" comes from the Greek *holos* which means whole. The term generally refers to the position that mind (soul) and body are one. Man is an inseparable unity. For the ancient Greeks, the psyche/soma unity was a life form. Today, a holistic approach means that mind and body are considered to be two distinct, yet integral aspects of the human being. More about this in Chap. 6".

[11] Dunbar herself had some misgivings about the term "psychosomatic interrelationships" as not doing justice to the fundamental unity of man.

The holistic approach, one of the most basic tenets of psychosomatic medicine, claims that man is an indivisible unity. Mind and body are abstractions from this unity. Not only is man a unity, man is also in constant interaction with his/her environment. However, when one examines the way "holism" functions in theory, it seems to be just another name for multi-factorial etiology, with unclear causality and limited efficacious mechanisms of interaction. Because of multi-factorial etiology and the division of man into a subjective realm of meaning, a material body and the environment, these theoreticians are forced to advocate an "inter-relation" between parts of an indivisible whole. Such a description has not furthered the understanding of psychosomatic pathology or given any comprehensible mechanisms of interaction, leaving the mind–body problem unsolved. The second conflict inherent in psychosomatic medicine is a clash between conflicting scientific interests, on the one hand, looking for nomothetic, universal laws[12] and at the same time embracing an open-ended idiographic approach, acknowledging the importance of the subjective meaning which persons' can ascribe to their situations. As a medical discipline, psychosomatic medicine needs quantified, experimental verification of its theoretical statements and wants to see at least some causal mechanisms. This strategy is not commensurable with the other major tenet of psychosomatic medicine, which acknowledges the importance of highly individualized, subjective factors in the creation of psychosomatic pathology. How can causal relations be established when such complex and almost endless combination of factors interact, such as the contribution of specific personality traits, coping skills, physiological make-up, social status, and finally, the individual meaning which a person ascribes to various life events and situations? This dilemma is not resolvable. If psychosomatic medicine wants to follow the natural sciences and formulate verified hypothesis and causal mechanisms, it cannot, at the same time, embrace the importance of qualitative, subjective meaning constitution of individuals in it the etiology of psychosomatic symptom formation. But if psychosomatic medicine gives up its vow to investigate the interrelation between the psychological and the physiological (found in "The Introductory Statement") it loses its *raison d'être,* as a special sub-discipline of medicine. Without taking into account individual, subjective, psychological, social factors in relation to health and illness and the interrelation between mind and body, psychosomatic medicine disintegrates into ordinary (somatic) medicine.

The problem with psychosomatic medicine, as with all materialistic psychosomatic theories is that theoreticians have a hard time defining the "psycho" in psycho-somatic. There has not been a great deal of interest in mind–body issues in

[12] For example Birley and Connolly (1976), "It is no longer good enough to predict" illness from "life-events" or to fail to do so. The aim should be to postulate certain mechanisms and then attempt to confirm or refute their existence by well-designed experiments" (p. 162) and Lipowsky (1976) "The task of psychosomatic research is to break down the enormous complexity of this interaction and formulate hypotheses about causal links and correlations among clearly defined and quantifiable variables" (p. 9).

psychosomatic medicine,[13] although there is some awareness that a stand must be taken on what one means by "the mental/psychological" in a discipline that has as its motto "[...] to study in their interrelation the psychological and physiological aspects of all normal and abnormal bodily functions and thus to integrate somatic therapy and psychotherapy" (Introductory Statement, *Journal of Psychosomatic Medicine,* 1:3). Graham's (1967) theory of linguistic parallelism is often referred to as a reasonable standpoint on the mind-body issue within this tradition. Linguistic parallelism states that the dualism which exists between mind and body is a *linguistic* dualism, based upon two different discourses of description, the physical and the mental. According to linguistic parallelism, different languages may be used to describe one and the same event. The mental and the physical are often thought of as referring to different types of events, but this is a mistake according to linguistic parallelism, there is only one event, described in different ways. The supposition behind this theory is that there exists a form of psycho-physical one to one correspondence between meaning constituting acts and brain processes. Psychosomatic medicine has no trouble in identifying what the body is (the physical, physiological side of the "parallelism"). However, it is more difficult to discern what is referred to by the psychological language? Brain processes are not experiences, nor can physiology give an adequate account of the psychological *as* psychological. The problem is subtle but clear. This theory places the material as primordial, as Graham states, "Patients can be thought of as having different aspects (psychological and physical), but any aspect is suitable for description in the somatic language, and many in the psychological" (p. 57).

Unfortunately, that which was to be the specialty of psychosomatic medicine, namely to study and explicate the nature of the *relationship* between the psychological and the physiological often gives way to the one-sided explication of physiology and neurological functioning. This can be seen as a misrepresentation of meaning as physiology, the same kind of error found in the examples from Solms in the previous section. Together with the biomedical model and the ideals of natural science, the "parallelism" between mind and body tends to slip into reductionism (the mind *is* merely the brain[14]).

Psychosomatic medicine is ambiguous on the mind-body issue. On the one hand, emphasis is placed upon the importance of psychological, social and

---

[13] For example Lipowsky who wrote that although psychosomatic medicine is concerned with investigating theories about bio-psycho-social relationships, "[...] while all this activity may be regarded as highly relevant to the debate about the mind–body problem, the latter cannot be viewed as the subject matter of psychosomatic medicine, which is an empirical and not a philosophical discipline" (1984), p. 168.

[14] A recent formulation of this confusion from Cameron (2001) "Thus, any theory that proposes to explain psychosomatic functions must involve an explanation of how the brain and the body interact, in both directions, how the brain affects the body and how the body affects the brain" (p. 697). The brain is of course a part of the body, not something other than the "stuff" that forms the rest of our materiality. The mind–body problem must be formulated in other terms, such as, how does meaning, volition and personhood relate to and affect the body? This is, of course, another question entirely.

physiological multi-factorial interdependence. No one description/language is said to be superior to another and using one language (the psychological or the physical) does not exclude using another language meaningfully about the same data. On the other hand, we find in linguistic parallelism a naturalistic bias which gives primordiality to physical descriptions. *Any observation whatsoever* can be described in physical terms, but necessarily the other way around.[15] If the psychological is capable, in principle, of being understood in physicalistic descriptions (neurons firing in the brain), one hardly has any need of psychosomatic medicine. However, if there is a dimension of human existence known as "the subjective", meaning, mind, signification (a dimension which is implied in the bio-psycho-social model espoused by psychosomatic medicine) which is not adequately described nor understood in the language of physiology, we should expect something more from psychosomatic medicine. Later research points out that the more popular science of "mind-body medicine" (Fava and Sonino 2000) has made key psychosomatic concepts more accessible to the public, but we are still caught up in the problem of how to understand the "interaction" between cells, tissues, organisms, and the personal subjective realm of existence. New concepts and variables have been introduced (recent life events, chronic stress and allostatic load, early life events, personality, psychological well-being, oriental alternative therapies and so on) but the inherent problems still remain. Six decades of psychosomatic medicine has not succeeded in providing a truly bio-psycho-social model of man nor providing comprehensible etiology nor causal relations.

> Despite much research effort, psychosomatic research has - from a medical point of view – in large been a disappointment. It has failed to produce knowledge to control any of the major health care problems [...] a large amount of empirical observations have accumulated, but the problem is that many of the findings cannot easily to related to one another (Jern and Carlsson 1990, p. 4:1).

Stress theory began as the investigation of the physiology of the stress reactions in laboratory rats subjected to various "stressors". Walter Cannon, considered the founding father of stress research, coined the term "homeostasis"[16] to describe the way the organism strives towards a state of stable equilibrium, although his research showed that the internal environment of the body was in fact seldom in a state of equilibrium. It was Hans Selye who would eventually develop the idea that the body's physiological reactions to provocations are an integral aspect of the stress reaction.

The modern, professional and academic understanding of stress is in line with our ordinary language usage, that is, stress is conceptualized as a relationship

---

[15] "All observations of people can be put in physical language terms, so that for any psychological statement whatever there may be a parallel physical statement. The reverse is not true [...]" Graham (1967), p. 56.

[16] "So as long as this personal, individual sack of salty water, in which each one of us lives and moves and has his being, is protected from change, we are freed from serious peril. Because that protection is afforded by special physiologic agencies, I have suggested that the stable state of the fluid matrix be given the name homeostasis." Cannon (1935), p. 2.

between the person and the environment which leads the person into a state of prolonged physiological arousal and cognitive dysfunction, eventually resulting in ill health. The stressed individual has appraised his/her relationship to the situation as taxing or exceeding his/her resources and, as a result, endangering his/her well-being. An important step forward in stress theory was the work of Lazarus and Folkman (1984), who opposed a simple stimulus–response conceptualization of stress and emphasized the importance of the *meaning* of the stressor for the person. When dealing with human beings (instead of rats) one must take into account the individuals' appraisal/understanding of the situation in order to understand the stress response. The meaning of a particular "stimulus" depends largely upon how that person has appraised the situation (as threatening or challenging, as manageable or not). What is stressful for one individual need not be stressful for another. All transactions with the environment are mediated by the meaning, signification or evaluation of the situation. The coping strategies available to a person will to a large degree determine if a situation is appraised as threatening or manageable. Interestingly, according to Lazarus, appraisal need not be conscious. A person may be unaware or unconscious of all the ideas, values and personal agendas which guide his or her understanding of a situation. This insight, although problematic in Lazarus' own theory (how can an appraisal, which seems to always be a cognitive judgment, be outside of awareness?) will be shown later on to make perfect sense from within a Merleau-Pontian perspective of the lived body.

What is the mind–body position implicit in stress theory? The philosophical question is rarely asked in the stress literature. However, a relevant version of the philosophical question would be, how does the experience of stress make one ill/diseased? Even here, not surprisingly, we find the role of the emotions to be central once again. Lazarus and Folkman (1984) write, "An essential theme of the analysis of stress, coping and health that dominates thinking in behavior medicine is that emotional states of all kinds and intensities accompany appraisals of harm, threat and challenge. The link with illness is the conventional one that massive bodily changes associated with emotions, especially strong, negative ones such as fear and anger." (p. 205). Emotions are not only tied to thoughts but bound up with a person's goals, commitment and values. According to Lazarus, the reason that emotions are relevant to stress theory is that they include components from psychology (affects, cognitions and value judgments), behavioral action impulses and physiological changes. The connection between emotion and ill health is the idea that repeated chronic emotional arousal is said to wear and tear on the system, leading ultimately to disease.[17] Although meaning is assumed to be an integral factor in understanding stress, there are no clear definitions about what meaning is. As in the previous theories, mind–body interaction is supposedly illustrated in the case of the emotions, which are said to build a bridge between meaning and physiology, although this

[17] Sometimes Lazarus seems to use the terms "emotion" and "stress" almost interchangeably. He has proposed that we should regard physiological stress as a subset of emotion, for example, "In fact, anger, anxiety, guilt, shame, sadness, envy, jealousy and disgust, which arise out of conflict, are commonly referred to as the stress emotions." (Lazarus 1993, p. 244).

bridge is never actually explicated. To put Lazarus in line with some classical philosophical position, he could in some sense be called a phenomenologist.[18] He is phenomenological in his thinking in the interest paid to the way in which individuals constitute the meaning of their situation. He is not phenomenological in any strict sense as he refers to the "objective world" showing that he has not implemented a phenomenological reduction. Nevertheless, there is a phenomenological thread in this approach which stands out in contrast to the previous theories.

If the underlying assumption that stress (as an experience) is related to coping and emotion is sound, how are we to understand the etiological mechanisms responsible for developing ill health? Cannon was not especially concerned with the question of stress-related disease, although he could imagine that chronic levels of the alarm response (fight or flight) might lead to a disruption of homeostasis, resulting in disturbed physiological functioning. It is first with the idea of *psychological* stress that one can begin to find some attempts to explicate this mechanism. According to Lazarus and Folkman, "Stress in itself is not a sufficient cause of disease. To produce stress-linked disease other conditions must also be present such as vulnerable tissue or coping processes that inadequately manage the stress. The primary task of research is to study the contribution of these other variables and processes as mediators of the stress-illness relationship." (1984, p. 18). We find once again a complex network of factors, comparable to the multi-factorial, open systems approach of psychosomatic medicine. The etiological components in stress theory as formulated by Lazarus are the following: (1) a potentially stressful (threatening) situation arising in the life of the individual (a situation understood here as a person-environment interaction), (2) an appraisal of the situation, containing not only conscious and unconscious thoughts, but also a matrix-like relationship of beliefs, commitments, emotions, motivations and goals, (3) coping skills and patterns, related to both personality traits and coping styles. Coping is furthermore conceptualized as a process, evolving over time, possibly even changing during the course of one and the same stressful event, (4) physiological reactions in the body, specifically catecholamine secretion, increased blood pressure, sharpened vigilance, energy mobilization with all that it physiologically entails, such as the secretion of glucocorticoids, which block the transport of nutrients into fat cells, the division of amino acids to the liver for immediate breakdown into glucose and so on. The mediating link between all these factors is appraisal. When a situation is appraised as stressful, and coping mechanisms are not available, the likely result is somatic disturbance, which can, if chronic, lead to disease. Thus, the explanation of efficacy (etiology) from mind to body rests upon the idea that sustained physiological arousal is detrimental to the organism, the same basic idea implicitly expressed in the theory of psychosomatic etiology found in the texts from psychosomatic medicine. Even if this would seem to make some sense, it is far from explaining all forms of psychosomatic symptoms.

[18] In one text Lazarus actually refers to "our phenomenology" (1984, p. 48) although he gives no phenomenological references.

Although the physiology of the stress-reaction has been mapped out, the link between stress as an experience and the ultimate development of ill health is not clear. What is the nature of the interaction between the meaning (appraisal) of the situation and the eventual development of disease? Do we really understand what coping is? The theoretical problems are similar to those found in psychosomatic medicine, namely, which factors interact with each other in what ways (and according to what mechanisms) in order to ultimately produce disease? Do we have a methodological problem here, i.e.—we just don't yet know all the factors involved, and although the picture is very complex, it is not incomprehensible—or are the difficulties surrounding the relationship between experience and meaning constitution and ill health in fact principle ones? My position is that we will never be able to produce the kind of explanatory links which both stress theory and psychosomatic medicine wish to see between the experience of stress, physiology, emotion, coping, beliefs, attitudes, behaviors and the development of disease and ill health. This cannot be done because these theories have broken up the natural unity of being-in-the world in order to comply with dualistic methodological strategies. How this particular life is lived and how this particular way of being-in-the world leads to a breakdown into psychosomatic symptoms and ill health demands a different type of inquiry. To understand why someone experiences stress in a certain situation and what it means to be in ill health requires a radically different way of conceiving of mind–body–world. This perspective is a phenomenological one which will be presented in the next chapter. But first, to complete the picture of the psychosomatic problematic, I will now briefly examine the clinical aspects of this dilemma.

The Clinical Challenges of Psychosomatic Pathology

The clinical challenges presented by psychosomatic health problems are four in number. Firstly, most health care organizations and methods of treatment are not amenable to this group of patients. Patients are expected to either have problems with the body, requiring somatic treatments like medication, surgery, traditional physiotherapy or problems with the mind, requiring psychological treatments such as psychotherapy and counseling. Since patients with psychosomatic symptoms have neither the one nor the other, strictly speaking, they find themselves in a no-man's land when they seek help. Secondly, the term "psychosomatic" is still perceived by many as a stigmatizing label implying that one is not really ill and somehow responsible for one's own ill health. The patient will often feel both shame and guilt, while the health care professionals may experience a variety of negative feelings towards these patients, ranging from mild irritation to contempt. Thirdly, the patient him/herself does not understand their ill health in terms of a psychosomatic problem, but rather as a particularly difficult somatic condition that no one seems to be able to cure. Finally, the cure in these cases is a time consuming process that requires a different approach to treatment than the traditional ones within somatic care and psychotherapy, respectively. All of these challenges result in non-productive clinical encounters, leaving both the patient and the health care professional frustrated and dissatisfied. Before I address each of these challenges in more detail, first to the question, how common are psychosomatic health problems?

Some studies show that up to a third of the physical symptoms that cause patients to seek primary health care are medically unexplainable (Kirmayer et al. 2004; Kroenke 1992). LÅTSTÅ there are some controversies surrounding the diagnosis and categorization of psychosomatic disorders (Wessely and White 2004) although some common characteristics have been found, such as over-representation of females, a history of negative early experiences, sudden onset, waxing and waning of the symptom, altered stress response (altered nervous system functioning during stressful periods) and resistance to therapeutic approaches (Buffington 2009). Persons who seek excessive medical attention, the so-called "frequent attenders" in primary care have traditionally been found to be female, older, less well educated, living with their spouses and/or children (Ferrai et al. 2008*)*. However, another study found that medically unexplained symptoms were over represented in younger females with employment (Nimnuan et al. 2001). There is thus no clear cut picture of who will develop psychosomatic symptoms although female overrepresentation and the failure of traditional treatments seem to be consistently found in the literature.

A five year study in the five Nordic countries investigating psychosomatic complaints in children aged 2–17 during 1984 and 1996 found that psychosomatic health problems have increased in all age groups, where socially and economically vulnerable families seemed to be a greater risk (Berntsson and Köhler 2001). A study from WHO (2008) showed that children's headaches, stomach pains, depressive thoughts and insomnia had almost doubled from 1985 to 2006. A 10 year study from Finland (Santalahi et al. 2005) also found that the prevalence of frequent headaches and abdominal pain amongst school aged children had increased from 1989 to 1999. In Japan, a large health questionnaire study showed that older schoolchildren were found to exhibit psychosomatic symptoms due to school difficulties and conflicts in interpersonal relationships (Tanaka et al. 2000). To conclude, there is sufficient empirical evidence to suggest that psychosomatic symptoms are the reason behind a substantial number of persons seeking health care, and there seems to be a trend pointing towards psychosomatic symptom formation in younger children and teenagers during the last few decades. If this is the case, it is imperative that we find acceptable treatments for these conditions, which means that we must gain a new understanding of what "psychosomatic" problems are all about. Let us just briefly examine the clinical challenges in greater detail.

The dualistic organization of health care is a major problem for these patients. There are some exceptions (like the Benson-Henry Institute for Mind Body Medicine in Massachusetts) but most traditional health care settings are still divided in terms of body or mind, having either professionals trained in the natural sciences (doctors and nurses) or professionals trained in the human sciences (psychologists, social workers, psychotherapists). Physiotherapists and occupational therapists, from the so-called rehabilitation professions, can be found in either camp, but are most often employed within somatically oriented health care institutions, working for example with rehabilitation after stroke, spinal cord injury, heart attacks, newly operated patients and the like.[19] In somatic health care, the human body is compartmentalized into medical sub-specializations such as the ear–nose–throat doctor, skin doctor, gynecologist, stomach–intestine doctor, the eye doctor, the neurologist, the cardiologist and so on, each subspecialty taking a part of the body as their area of competence. The psychotherapeutic services are comprised mostly of different forms of "talking cures" although sometimes non-verbal therapy forms are available, such as dance therapy, music therapy or art therapy. However, the patient who has psychosomatic complaint will not seek psychotherapy or counseling since s/he experiences problems with their body, so the first appointment will most probably be made with the General Practitioner in primary care. Depending upon the complaint, the first line of treatment will be medication or physical therapy, sometimes laboratory tests are taken if the doctor is not sure of a diagnosis or line of treatment. When the initial treatments (medication, physical therapy) prove to be ineffective, it is time for the next round. Further tests are then taken, where new medications or a referral to a specialist may be the next step. By this time the patient has become anxious and distressed since the symptom has not abated and the health care professionals have no explanation as to why the treatment is not working. Anxiety and worry exacerbate the symptom, so the patient feels worse the further s/he progresses into the health care system. At this point, the scenario changes from the normal "liturgy of the clinic",[20] and the patient begins to experience his/herself as a deviant. The health care professionals may start to see the patient as a "problem" patient. Depending upon the way in which the patient is treated, s/he may become hostile and aggressive towards the health care professionals, not trusting them nor believing in their efforts to find a cure. When the patient's trust and confidence has been damaged in this way, it impedes any moving forward in the therapeutic process. There is a risk that the patient will become locked in defensiveness and aggression, and without the cooperation of the patient, it will be impossible to find a cure.

There is still a great deal of stigmatization associated with the term "psychosomatic" patient, despite the awareness today of mind–body issues and the advent of mind–body medicine. In previous times, before we had any understanding of mind–body issues, persons with psychosomatic conditions were perceived as having no "real" health problems and were considered to be malingerers or lazy, trying to get out of work or responsibilities by pretending to be ill. But if we have a better understanding of psychosomatics today, why is the term still so degrading?

---

[19] An exception to this is PTs and OTs working within psychiatric care and specialized pain clinics. In these areas, the rehabilitation staff is often integrated in a multi-professional team, where s/he may work with different forms of non-verbal therapy which can be beneficial for patients with psychosomatic conditions who have initial problems with reflection and verbalization. More on this in Chap. 5.

[20] See Mishler (1984).

One reason is the dualistic organization of health care described above. If our conceptualization of health problems were not dualistic, persons with these kinds of problems would not feel stigmatized. They would be treated like any other patient at the clinic or on the ward, even if their problems did not neatly fit into the category "problems of the body" or "problems of the mind". If health care professionals felt confident and competent with these patients, the patient would not feel stigmatized. If health care professionals had a better understanding of the psychosomatic process and pedagogical ways of discussing psychosomatics with the patient, as well as a repertoire of efficacious treatment strategies, the patient would not feel stigmatized.

Why is it necessary to "educate" the patient about psychosomatics? The reason is because the patient has, for various reasons, designated the place of his/her suffering in the body. How we can understand this level of expression will be discussed in Chap. 5. For now, suffice to say that had the person been able to handle their life situation with thoughts, feelings and actions, it would not have been necessary to develop the symptom. The key to a successful psychosomatic treatment is that the patient must let go of the body (psychosomatic) solution and become open, at least on an intellectual level, to the idea that the body symptoms are a reaction to something going on in his/her life. This "psychosomatic turn" will not occur on its own, since the psychosomatic solution is the only way the person knows how to cope when they seek help. Bad health care encounters can also sediment hostility towards health care professionals and produce a negative reaction to any suggestions that the problem is not in the body, but "in the head." In order to re-define the health problem, the patient must be willing to accept that the answer to their problems does not lie in further medical treatment. The stigmatization of having psychosomatic problems must be lifted and this can only happen through respectful dialogue with the health care professional who can explain to the patient that they are not crazy or malingerers, but simply overwhelmed to the point that their body is trying to do the work that they should be doing on another level in order to deal with their life situation. Patients have often rejected their bodies and also need help in order to regain care and respect for the "thing" that is giving them so much trouble. All of this work needs to be done first, before an actual treatment can begin.

The last clinical challenge is the time consuming nature of the treatment, which may even involve several different health care professionals (a medical doctor, a nurse, a physiotherapist, a psychologist). In psychiatric care and specialized pain clinics it is not unusual to find multi-professional teams, but in primary care, where these patients first show up, this is generally not the case. Patients exhibiting these kinds of symptoms require other professional skills, competence and health care organization than patients who have either somatic- or psychological health problems. For this reason, a deeper understanding of this group of patients also means we need to examine how primary care is organized and look critically at how the education and training of health care professionals treats the "psychosomatic". In the following chapters, this alternative understanding, based upon a phenomenological perspective, will be presented both in terms of theory and practice.

References

Alexander, F. (1939). Introductory Statement to. *Psychosomatic Medicine, 1939*(1), 1.

Barsky, A. J., Orav, E. J., & Bates, D. W. (2005). Somatization increases medical utilization and costs independent of psychiatric and medical comorbidity. *Archives of General Psychiatry, 62*, 903–910.

Berntsson, L. T., & Köhler, L. (2001). Long-term illness and psychosomatic complaints in children aged 2–17 years in the five Nordic countries: Comparison between 1984–1996. *European Journal of Public Health, 11*(1), 35–42.

Birley, J. L. T., & Connolly, J. (1976). Life events and physical illness. In O. Hill (Ed.), *Modern trends in psychosomatic medicine, 3* (pp. 154–165). London: Butterworths.

Buffington, C. A. T. (2009). Developmental influences on medically unexplained symptoms. *Psychotherapy and Psychosomatics, 78*, 139–144.

Bynum, W. F., & Porter, R. (Eds.). (1993). *The role of emotional factors in somatic disease in companion encyclopedia of the history of medicine* (Vol. 2). London: Routledge.

Cameron, O. (2001). Introception: The inside story—a model for psychosomatic processes. *Psychosomatic Medicine, 63*, 697–710.

Cannon, W. (1935). The stresses and strains of homeostasis. *American Journal of Medical Sciences, 189*, 1–14.

Cederqvist, Å. V. (2006). Psychiatric and psychosomatic symptoms are increasing problems among Swedish schoolchildren. *Acta Paediatrica, 95*, 901–903.

Denollet, J. (2005). DS14: Standard assessment of negative affectivity, social inhibition, and type D personality. *Psychosomatic Medicine, 67*(1), 89–97.

Deutsch, F. (1959). *On the mysterious leap from the mind to the body: A workshop study on the theory of conversion*. New York: International Universities Press, Inc.

Dunbar, F. (1935). *Emotions and bodily changes, a survey of literature on psychosomatic interrelationships*. New York: Columbia University Press.

Fava, A. G., & Sonino, N. (2000). Psychosomatic medicine: Emerging trends and perspectives. *Psychotherapy and Psychosomatics, 69*, 184–197.

Ferrai, S., Galeazzi, G. M., Mackinnon, A., & Rigatelli, M. (2008). Frequent attenders in primary care: Impact of medical, psychiatric and psychosomatic diagnoses. *Psychotherapy and Psychosomtics, 77*, 306–314.

Fink, P., Toft, T. Hansen M. S., et al, (2005) Classification of somatization and functional somatic symptoms in primary care. *Australian and New Zealand Journal of Psychiatry*, 39, 772–781.

Freud, S. (1909). Notes upon a case of obsessional neurosis. *Standard edition of the complete works of Sigmund Freud* (vol. X). London: The Hogarth Press.

Freud, S. (1915). Papers on metapsychology. *Standard edition of the complete works of Sigmund Freud* (vol. XIV). London: The Hogarth Press.

Freud, S. (1938/1940). An outline of psycho-analysis. *Standard edition of the complete works of Sigmund Freud,* (vol. XIII). London: The Hogarth Press.

Graham, D. T. (1967). Health, disease, and the mind-body problem: Linguistic parallelism. *Psychosomatic Medicine, 29*, 52–71.

Jellesma, F. C. (2008). Health in young people: Social inhibition and negative affect and their relationship with self-reported somatic complaints. *Journal of Developmental and Behavioral Pediatrics, 29*(2), 94–100.

Jern, S. & Carlsson, S. G. (1990). Metatheory of psychosomatic research. *Gothenburg Psychological Reports* No 4, Vol 20.

Kirmayer, L. J., Groleau, D., Looper, K. J., & Dominicé, M. (2004). Explaining medically unexplained symptoms. *The Canadian Journal of Psychiatry/La Revue canadienne de psychiatrie, 49*(10), 663–672.

Kroenke, K. (1992). Symptoms in medical patients: An unattended field. *American Journal of Medicine, 92*, 3–6.

Lazarus, R. (1993). Coping theory and research: Past, present and future. *Psychosomatic Medicine, 55*, 234–247.
Lazarus, R., & Folkman, S. (1984). *Stress, appraisal and coping*. New York: Springer Publishing Co.
Lipowsky, Z. J. (1976). Psychosomatic Medicine: an Overview. In O. Hill (Ed.), *Modern trends in psychosomatic medicine 3* (pp. 1–20). London: Butterworths.
Lipowsky, Z. J. (1984). What does the word "psychosomatic" really mean? A historical and semantic inquiry. *Psychosomatic Medicine, 46*, 153–171.
Mason, J. W. (1975). Emotions as reflected in patterns of endocrine integration. In L. Levi (Ed.), *Emotions: Their parameters and measurement*. New York: Raven.
MacDougall, J. (1985). *Theatres of the mind: Truth and illusion on the psychoanalytic stage*. Great Brittan: Brunner-Routledge.
MacDougall, J. (1989). *Theaters of the body: A psychoanalytic approach to psychosomatic illness*. New York: Norton.
Magretts, E. L. (1954). Historical notes on psychosomatic medicine. In E. D. Wittkower & R. A. Cleghorn (Eds.), *Recent developments in psychosomatic medicine*. London: Sir Isaac Pitman & Sons Ltd.
Mishler, E. (1984). *The discourse of medicine: Dialectics of medical interview*. Norwood: Ablex.
Nimnuan, C., Hotopf, M., & Wessely, S. (2001). Medically unexplained symptoms: An epidemiological study in seven specialities. *Journal of Psychosomatic Research, 51*(1), 361–367.
Ormel, J. Von, Korff, M., Ustun, B., Pini, S., Korten, A., & Oldehinkel, T. (1994). Common mental disorders and disability across cultures. *JAMA, 272*, 1741–1748.
Pedersen, S. S., & Denollet, J. (2006). Is Type D personality here to stay? Emerging evidence across cardiovascular disease patient groups. *Current Cardiology Reviews, 2*, 205–213.
Ricoeur, P. (1970). *Freud and philosophy: An essay on interpretation*. New Haven: Yale University Press.
Royal College of Physicians, Royal College of Psychiatrists (2003). *The psychological care of medical patients. A practical guide* (1st ed.). Report of a Joint Working Party. London: Royal College of Physicians.
Santalahi, P., Aromaa, M., Sourander, A., Helenius, H., & Piha, J. (2005). Have there been changes in children's psychosomatic symptoms? A 10-year comparison from Finland. *Pediatrics, 2005*(115), e434. doi:10.1542/peds.2004-1261.
Solms, M. (1997). What is consciousness? *Journal of the American Psychoanalytic Association, 45*, 681–703.
Solms, M., & Turnbull, O. (2002). *The brain and the inner world*. New York: Other Press.
Tanaka, H., Tamai, H., Terashima, S., Takenaka, Y., & Tanaka, T. (2000). Psychological factors affecting psychosomatic symptoms in Japanese schoolchildren. *Pediatrics International, 42*, 354–358.
Wessely, S., & White, P. D. (2004). There is only one functional somatic syndrome. *British Journal of Psychiatry, 185*, 95–96.
World Health Organization (2008). Inequalities in young people's health, Health behaviour in school-aged children (HBSC), ISBN 978 92890 7195 6.

Chapter 2
The Lived Body

Phenomenology

The philosopher Maurice Merleau-Ponty (1908–1961) is an important thinker within the phenomenological tradition although his life has not been as exposed and analyzed as for example Sartre or Foucault.[1] He attended the prestigious *Ècole Normal Superior*, where he studied together with Jean-Paul Sartre and Simone de Beauvoir. His *docteur des lettre* (doctoral dissertation) was comprised of his first two philosophical works, *The Structure of Behavior* (1942/1963) and *Phenomenology of Perception* (1945/1962). In this dissertation, he formulated his understanding of phenomenology as a "way of thinking" and worked out a groundbreaking view of the body and the importance of the body for philosophy. But before I present this work, an introduction to phenomenology is needed in order to fully understand Merleau-Ponty's philosophical contribution.

Phenomenologists often spend the first third of their work explaining what phenomenology is not. True to that tradition, let me begin by explaining what phenomenologists call "the natural attitude", which is our everyday way of seeing and understanding the world around us. This taken-for-granted, everyday understanding of the world is shot through with ideas, pre-understanding and prejudices which very seldom come to light, since it is "natural" to not examine them.[2] However, these ideas and pre-suppositions stand in the way of the subject matter of phenomenology, which is the systematic study of the realm of subjectivity. Phenomenology *does not* study the objective world as such, but rather the subjective foundations for being able to experience the world as objective and independent of our acts of attending and understanding. The way in which the world appears (shows itself) to human beings in and through subjectivity (consciousness) is the focus of phenomenology. The founder of phenomenology,

[1] See Carman 2008; Diprose and Reynolds 2008; Hass 2008 for litterature on Merleau-Ponty's philosophy with some biographical material.
[2] The un-problematized belief in the reality of the world is also called the thetic/positional/existential/ontic reality character of perception. Ricoeur has poetically called this positing of realness as "the vehemence of presence."

J. Bullington, *The Expression of the Psychosomatic Body from a Phenomenological Perspective*, SpringerBriefs in Philosophy,
DOI: 10.1007/978-94-007-6498-9_2,

Edmund Husserl, called subjectivity "the wonder of all wonders". It is the very ground for all our experience and knowledge and is the medium through which we can have contact with the world which we call "reality." Phenomenology does not doubt the existence of the world, it simply recognizes that this certainty is yet another non-examined belief (part of the natural attitude) and as such must be examined in terms of subjectivity, which is the pre-condition for all knowledge and understanding. There are two very different epistemologies (theories of knowledge) underlying the natural attitude, with its belief in the objective reality of the world, and phenomenology, which takes its point of departure in the subjective. I will just briefly present these two points of view.

The objectivistic point of view could be characterized as "the view from nowhere" (Nagel 1989). This perspective could also be called a God's eye view, where it is assumed that there exists an independent reality that can be correctly described in symbolic representations (language) which correspond to things and relationships in the "real world." According to the objectivistic view, there is a neutral perspective beyond human limitations, independent of human subjectivity and embodiment, a transcendent "objective" stance outside of the relationship person-world, in which the alleged correspondence between things and what-is-said-about-things can be judged. Knowledge is objective, in the sense that it can be verified as factual states of affairs in the real world. The ideal of objectivity is one of the most cherished and prominent characteristics of natural science. The notion of a subject-independent reality is so ingrained in our cultural thinking that it is difficult to imagine knowledge and meaning in any other way. But however useful this idea may be in other contexts, it prevents us from grasping the subjective ground of thinking and understanding. In order to study the subjective in a positive way, and not merely as a disturbing interfering variable, we need an alternative way of thinking about the subjective. Phenomenology can reveal this dimension by the adoption of a different stance than the objectivistic one.

Phenomenology is the philosophical movement in Continental philosophy stemming from the works of Edmund Husserl (1913/1962; 1954/1970). The term "phenomenology" means literally the *logos* (or inherent meaning or order) of phenomena, that is to say, the meaning of that which appears or shows itself to man. How human beings perceive, understand and live the world is the subject matter of phenomenological study. Again, it is the realm of subjectivity that is the focus of interest for phenomenology. Husserl's life project was to establish phenomenology as a rigorous science, on a par with the natural sciences that studied nature (the world of things). However, since the subject matter for phenomenology differed in kind from the subject matter of the natural sciences, Husserl had to create a methodology and concepts that would be suitable for the study of human "meaning constitution", to use another term. He understood that the objective methodologies, so successful in natural science, would not do justice to the subjective.[3] The study of “appearances” would need a new approach. This approach was worked out in Husserl’s phenomenological thinking and gave inspiration to an entire phenomenological movement.[4]

One can for the sake of simplicity, summarize the radical change in perspective from the objective view of the natural sciences to the phenomenological interest in subjectivity as a shift of focus. Instead of studying the world of objects in the material world, as the natural scientist does, phenomenologists, having decided to study another realm, place the “real” objective world in brackets, performing the so-called *epoché*, or phenomenological reduction. The term “reduction” by no means implies reducing wholes to parts or looking for the least common denominator, but comes from the latin *re-ducere*, which means “to lead back”. Husserl’s use of the term reduction as *re-ducere* was a call to return to the things themselves, that is, to the way in which the world shows itself in and through consciousness, in order to obtain knowledge about the subjective realm. The phenomenological reduction places the reality status of the world and the objective qualities of things within brackets (suspends our taken-for-granted belief in them) in order to concentrate on an area that is non-thematic and impossible to see as long as the objective perspective is dominant.

By putting aside all interest in the existence of the real world and the objective qualities of things, phenomenology shifted focus to the manner of appearance, that is, to the way in which human consciousness attends to that which appears *as* it appears to consciousness. The focus of interest is how things present themselves (manner of presentation) and how consciousness “constitutes” the meaning of that which appears. This meaning constitution is discovered by examining the streaming of consciousness towards that which is outside of consciousness. The technical term for the streaming of consciousness towards something outside of itself is “intentionality”. Intentionality is a term Husserl borrowed from Brentano (1982), characterizing the way in which consciousness always points towards or “intends” its objects (“object” here referring to that *towards which* consciousness flows). In order to study the way in which consciousness intends or constitutes its object, the reality status of the world must be put aside. This does not mean that phenomenologists deny the existence of the real world, as mentioned before, it merely announces another focus of interest, requiring its own methods and terminology. Working out this philosophical strategy was Husserl’s life project.

---

3 This insight was also formulated already by Dilthey in the 1800s. Dilthey, the father of the so-called “human sciences” is known for the motto, “nature we explain, the life of the soul we understand.” The point here being that the methodologies used and results obtained from the natural sciences (causal, nomothetic type of knowledge) are not appropriate to the study of man. Terms like “meaning”, “value”, “signification” and “motivation” would be appropriate terms to use when studying man, according to Dilthey, rather than the objectivistic language used to describe things in nature.

4 See Spiegelberg (1982) for a comprehensive overview of the phenomenological movement.

A common misunderstanding about phenomenology is that the study of "appearances" would be less important than the study of the real world. An appearance is, after all, merely an appearance, less viable than real things, certainly secondary in importance to the study of real transcendent objects. We tend to give natural-scientific descriptions of things a higher status than the world we experience through our senses. However, as Husserl (1954/1970) pointed out, the world we experience is in fact primordial, that is to say, prior to natural-scientific descriptions of the world. We saw round objects in the world before this experience became abstracted into the mathematical concept of the circle. We saw how grains of sand make up a continuous stretch of beach before we started to construct theories about particles and atoms. According to Husserl, it is precisely on the basis of lived experience (i.e. "appearances") that we have been able to construct the abstract terminology and explanations conceptualized by natural science. Unfortunately, according to Husserl (1954/1970) we have forgotten this grounding of science in the primordial experience of the world, and this forgetting has resulted in the depreciation of the so-called "life-world." Life-world (*Lebenswelt*) refers to the everyday world of common experience. We find ourselves immersed in the life-world, consisting of values, beliefs, assumptions and cultural practices. The life-world is the unproblematic, pre-scientific world that constitutes the meaning of everyday life. Phenomenology affirms the life-world and the study of appearances as vital areas of study.

To reiterate, phenomenology does not make statements about how the world is in-itself, outside of human beings experiences of it. The subject matter of phenomenological studies is an examination of various human phenomena such as for example, perception, time consciousness, sexuality, religious and cultural practices, the body, the experience of the Holy etc. from the point of view of meaning constitution. In order to study these phenomena, it is necessary to implement the phenomenological reduction (bracket the reality character of the world) and focus upon the world-as-meant, or world-as-intended. When we do this, we find, according to Husserl, two poles of experience, one of which corresponds to the streaming of consciousness (*noesis* or noetic acts) and the other of which corresponds to that which consciousness attends to (*noema* or noematic objects). In place of the objective "real" object we find, under the phenomenological reduction, the streaming of consciousness towards the object-as-meant. This bracketed realm of *noesis* and *noema* is the study proper of phenomenology. It would be outside of the scope of this chapter to give a detailed account of the phenomenological method and the various forms of the phenomenological reduction. In this context it will suffice to say that phenomenology comprises an alternative to objectivistic epistemology, an alternative that takes its starting point in how the world appears to human beings. Within this perspective, we may now turn to Merleau-Ponty's philosophical reflection upon the body.

Merleau-Ponty's Phenomenology

Merleau-Ponty had a good idea of what he wanted to accomplish already as a young doctoral student. At the age of 25 he turned in two research proposals that contained the themes he would come to work with in his first two philosophical texts, *The Structure of Behavior* from 1942 and *Phenomenology of Perception* from 1945. The focus of these two works was a phenomenological reflection on the nature of perception and human embodiment. Later on in his career he turned his attention to a variety of other topics, such as language acquisition (1964/1973), expression and meaning (1960/1964) and literature and art (1948/1964; 1969/1973), but his interest in perception and the body remained with him throughout his career. His last work *The Visible and the invisible,* published posthumously in 1964 from his working notes, was a return to the theme of human embodiment and the relationship between mind–body and world. Many have read this last work as a critique of his earlier work and as an important step towards a new ontology. His concept "flesh of the world" from *The Visible and the Invisible* (1964/1968) was meant to describe the *event* where perception and meaning are born, not as a relationship between a constituting subject and a constituted object (traditional phenomenology) but as an intertwining or ensemble of being. In this last work he questioned the privileged position given to consciousness within phenomenology and maintained that we need to find another way to investigate the human world. The development of Merleau-Ponty's thought in this later work will be examined in Chap. 4. For now, we may simply note that he spent his entire philosophical career reflecting on the nature embodiment and how embodied human beings experience the world.

Merleau-Ponty shows in his first two works how many of our ideas about the human body and the nature of perception are conditioned by notions and concepts from natural science. These notions make it hard for us to reflect upon and discover how we experience our bodies in the world, and how we experience the world through our bodies. We understand perception, for example, in terms of stimuli-response. Although we never experience a stimulus, we are convinced that sight (visual perception), for example, is "really" all about light waves hitting the occipital lobe in the brain. This is, of course, a perfectly legitimate way to describe vision from within a certain perspective, but it is not the way we *live* seeing the world. If we only focus upon chemical, neurological processes, we miss the way in which the experience and meaning of the world unfolds for us. Human experience is the result of a unique relation between the embodied subject and that which shows itself to him/her at every instant. The subject and the world are "born together" (the word for knowledge in French is *conaissance*, which means literally, born together) in a movement that has been poorly understood by both science and philosophy.[5] We need to bracket our everyday notions about the objective body and natural-scientific notions about the nature of perception in order to elucidate the "dialogue" between the subject and his/her world.

How then to disclose this uncharted territory? Merleau-Ponty begins by assuring us that there is certainly something outside of ourselves which we are born into, which we have no choice but to relate to in one way or another. This "something" is present to us in ways that we experience through our senses. But this world outside ourselves is not imprinted upon us like a photograph, but taken up in an active moment of meaning constitution. Merleau-Ponty describes this meeting in the following way:

> Thus a sensible datum which is on the point of being felt sets a kind of muddled problem for my body to solve. I must find the attitude which *will* provide it with the means of becoming determinate, of showing up as blue; I must reply to a question which is obscurely expressed. And yet I do so only when I am invited by it, my attitude is never sufficient to make me really see blue or really touch a hard surface [...] As I contemplate the blue of the sky I am not set over against it as an a-cosmic subject; I do not possess it in thought, or spread out towards it some idea of blue such as might reveal the secret of it, I abandon myself to it and plunge into this mystery, it 'thinks itself within me'..." (p. 214, italics in original) and, "Apart from the probing of my eye or my hand, and before my body synchronizes with it, the sensible is nothing but a vague beckoning" (1945/1962, p. 214).

The classical subject-object dichotomy is loosened up and we find an area "between" subject and object, and it is only within this middle ground that the experience of what we call the world can arise. To take an illustrative example, imagine the phenomenon of figure/ground, a well-known principle from Gestalt psychology. I may look outside the window to see if my friend has arrived, or I may change perspective and notice that the window is dirty and needs to be cleaned. Foreground and background only exist between a subject who meets a view with certain interests and attention, and a world that shows itself *in terms of the* subject's interests and attention.[6] We cannot see both the smudge on the window and the friend coming up the drive at the same time, as illustrated by the famous perceptual example of from Gestalt psychology of the vase and the two faces. One can only see the vase or the faces, never both at the same time. Both are *there* simultaneously in the picture (objectively), but only available perceptually (subjectively) one at a time. That which is present perceptually is thus dependent upon the subject. However, the subject needs to be given the opportunity to orient himself/herself towards the dirty window or the friend, the vase or the two faces. One sees only what one is "invited" to see, as Merleau-Ponty expresses it.

---

[5] "We must rediscover, as anterior to the ideas of subject and object, the fact of my subjectivity and the nascent object, that primordial layer at which both things and ideas come into being." (1945/1962), p. 219.

[6] See Bredlau (2011) for a Merleau-Pointian account of the figure/ground structure of sense experience.

The phenomenon of figure/ground is a striking example of something that is constitutive of perception itself, namely, that there is always a given perspective in perception since there is always an embodied subject. The world is there *for me*, even if it is also an inter-subjective arena where I share my "view" with others, who have their own "views". Our mistake has been to lose sight of this relationship and divide up experience in terms of an objective world, understood in terms of natural science, and an objective, anonymous body that processes various stimuli in the brain. But the world is not an objective collection of things lying about, and the human body is not a processing machine. Again, this description is entirely correct if we wish to study the world from an objectivistic point of view, but here the interest is in phenomenology and the study of the subjective, so we put aside this naturalistic conceptualization and examine experience in terms of subjectivity, embodiment and meaning constitution. If we disregard the subject-object dichotomy and focus upon the realm of the "in-between", we will discover a lived unity that we could call a mind–body unity always present to the world, in one way or another. The "world", again, should be understood as the dialogue between the embodied human being and the presentation of something which beckons to us as an invitation to understand. Merleau-Ponty (1945/1962) writes, "Inside and outside are inseparable. The world is wholly inside and I am wholly outside of myself." (p. 407) and "The world is not what I think, but what I live through. I am open to the world, I have no doubt that I am in communication with it, but I do not possess it; it is inexhaustible." (ibid, pp. 16–17).

The Body and the World (Lived Body)

Merleau-Ponty calls the lived unity of the mind–body-world system "the lived body".[7] The body understood as a *lived body* is necessarily ambiguous, since it is both material and self-conscious. It is physiological and psychological, but Merleau-Ponty asserts that these terms are not as dichotomous as one would imagine. There is mind in the body and body in the mind.

> [...] The psycho-physical event can no longer be conceived after the model of Cartesian physiology and as the juxtaposition of a process in itself [the body] and a *cogitatio* [the mind]. The union of soul and body is not an amalgamation between two mutually external terms, subject and object, brought about by arbitrary degree. It is enacted at every instant in the movement of existence (1945/1962, pp. 88–89).
>
> It is impossible to superimpose on man a lower layer of behavior which one chooses to called "natural" followed by a manufactured cultural or spiritual world. Everything is both

[7] Translated from the French *le corps propre,* which means literally owns own body, the actual body, the pure/clean body. Sometimes the term *le corps vivant* is used as well, which translates as "the living body". The distinction between the objective and lived body was described in Husserl as a differentiation between the body's thing like aspects *(körper)* from the intentional, living aspects *(Leib).*

> manufactured and natural in man, as it were, in the sense that there is not a word, not a form of behavior which does not owe something to purely biological being – and which at the same time does not elude the simplicity of animal life, and cause forms of vital behavior to deviate from their pre-ordained direction, through a sort of *leakage* and through a genius for ambiguity which might serve to define man (ibid, p. 189).

These realms are to be understood as levels, intertwined with each other, constituting a unified field. The self, the body and the world of things and others are neither separated from each other nor to be confused with each other, but rather can be seen as three sectors or levels of a unique field. The lived body is always oriented towards the world outside itself (otherness) in a constant flow. In order to understand what this means, let us examine in detail what Merleau-Ponty writes about the body.

Merleau-Ponty is sometimes called "the philosopher of the body." He was not the first phenomenologist to draw attention to the body, Husserl had already written about the body as *Leib*,[8] but Merleau-Ponty placed the ambiguity of the body, as materiality and consciousness at the center of his philosophical investigation. The body Merleau-Ponty investigates and describes is not the objective body, in its materiality, but the subjective, lived body, in its constant "dialogue" with the world. To give an idea of the special status of the human body, let us listen to Merleau-Ponty's own voice:

> It is particularly true that an object is an object insofar as it can be moved away from me and ultimately disappear from my field of vision. Its presence is such that it entails a possible absence. Now the permanence of my own body is entirely different in kind: it is not at the extremity of some indefinite exploration; it defies exploration and is always presented to me from the same angel. Its permanence is not a permanence in the world, but a permanence on my part. To say that it is always near me, always there for me, is to say that it is never really in front of me, I cannot array it before my eyes, that it remains marginal to all my perceptions, that it is *with* me. It is true that external objects too never turn one of their sides to me without hiding the rest, but I can at least freely choose the side which they are to present to me (1945/1962, pp. 90–91).
>
> In so far as it sees or touches the world, my body can therefore be neither seen nor touched. What prevents its ever being an object [...] is that it is that by which there are objects. It is neither tangible nor visible in so far as it is that which sees and touches. The body therefore is not one more among external objects, with the peculiarity of always being there. If it is permanent, the permanence is absolute and is the ground for the relative permanence of disappearing objects [...] (ibid, p. 92).
>
> True reflection presents me to myself not as an idle and inaccessible subjectivity, but as identical with my presence in the world and to others, as I am now realizing it: I am all that I see, I am an intersubjective field, not despite my body and historical situation, but on the contrary, by being this body and this situation, and through them, all the rest (ibid, p. 452).
>
> We said earlier that it is the body which "understands" in the acquisition of habit. This way of putting it will appear absurd, if understanding is subsuming a sense-datum under an idea, and if the body is an object. But the phenomenon of habit is just what prompts us to revise our notion of "understand" and our notion of the body. To understand is to

---

[8] Merleau-Ponty has even said that his philosophy can be seen as drawing out "the un-thought thought" already present in Husserl's work.

experience the harmony between what we aim at and what is given, between the intention and the performance – and the body is our anchorage in the world (ibid, p. 144).

My body is the fabric into which all objects are woven [...] (ibid, p. 235).

My body is the pivot of the world: I know that objects have several facets because I could make a tour of inspection of them, and in that sense I am conscious of the world through the medium of my body (ibid, 82).

These quotes illustrate the insight that the lived body cannot be understood apart from the system "mind–body–world." Where there is a body, there is a personal world, an opening upon the world which is unique. This uniqueness has to do with our life as mind, as persons, with the fact that we have language, history and culture and can ask questions about our own existence. Likewise, there is no personal life or mind without a body, even though the science fiction genre often plays with the trope of a disembodied head kept alive in a jar, as in the film *Cold Lazarus*, or a body without a soul, as in the multitude of films about zombies. Finally, this intertwined mind–body-presence is always embedded in a concrete situation. There is no world (as perceived) without a human to experience it, and there is no human experience that is not of the world. Thus, we cannot discuss the body as if it were something cut off from both mind and world.

How does Merleau-Ponty tackle the so-called mind–body problem? He wants to retain dualism, but a "good" dualism that acknowledges a realm of human signification that cannot be reduced to or understood in terms of materiality. But dualism is traditionally riddled with "interaction" problems. In order retain the realm of mind without winding up in dualisms classical problems, the conceptualization of mind and body needs to be reformulated. Already in his first work, *Structure of Behavior*, he wrote:

[...] the notions of soul and mind must be revitalized; there is the body as a mass of chemical components in interaction, the body as a dialectic of lived being and its biological milieu, and the body as a dialectic of a social subject and his group... The body in general is an ensemble of paths already traced out, of powers already constituted; the body is the acquired dialectic soil upon which a higher "formation" is accomplished, and the soul is the meaning which is then established (1942/1963, p. 210).

[...] the relations of the soul and body – obscure as long as the body is treated in abstraction as a fragment of matter – are clarified when one sees the body as a bearer of a dialectic (ibid, 204).

Merleau-Ponty wanted to bring the body into phenomenology as a constituting subject (not a constituted thing), which meant he had to clear phenomenology of Husserl's bias of consciousness as the center of subjectivity. Merleau-Ponty points out that we are always already this being who is both mind and body in a natural unity. Mind and body are not the same, but neither are they as distinct from one another as Cartesian dualism has led us to believe.[9] Merleau-Ponty prefers to speak of "planes of signification" rather than different sorts of being or different orders

[9] "The ego as a center from which his intentions radiate, the body which carries them and the beings and things to which they are addressed are not confused, but they are only three sectors of a unique field." (1942, p. 189).

of reality. The discussion of how material physiological processes relate to meaning (the human psycho-social realm) is both fascinating and insoluble. Merleau-Ponty comments in *Phenomenology of Perception,* "How significance and intentionality could come to dwell in molecular edifices or masses in cells is a thing which can never be made comprehensible, and here Cartesianism is right. But there is, in any case, no question of any such absurd undertaking." (p. 201). The mind–body problem has its origin in faulty conceptualizations of both mind and body. The "objective" material body is already intentional and fully engaged in meaning constitution (the body "knows" things below the level of consciousness) and the mind is through and through an incarnated mind. These levels are naturally intertwined as human embodiment. This is the way we are in the world. This mind/body unity is likewise always relating to a concrete lived situation (called "the world"). Merleau-Ponty embraces both the life of the "soul" (mind) as well as the reality of our corporeal existence, tied inextricably to our body. The physiology and materiality of the body are indispensable in that they set the frame for our possibilities, but we are never causally determined by our physical being.[10] Our concrete existence as beings who live in a meaningful world is never the product or result of physiological processes. We are also psychological, cultural beings. The materiality of our body is a fundament which is taken up and transformed into levels of existence which lie over and above our brute physicality.[11]

If the mind and body are not distinct regions for Merleau-Ponty, understood in diametrical opposition to one another, which is their relationship? One could say that the mental and the physical overlap or intertwine. We are always both mind and body, but different levels of our being (mental or physical) are evoked to a greater or less degree by different situations, giving us a picture of movement on a mind–body continuum. This "movement" is characterized in the following way:

> Man taken as a concrete being is not just a psyche joined to an organism, but the movement to and fro of existence which at one time allows itself to take corporeal form

---

[10] In *Structure of Behavior* Merleau-Ponty writes of the painter El Greco: "If one supposes an anomaly of vision in El Greco, as has sometimes been done, it does not follow that the form of the body in his paintings, and consequently the style of the attitudes, admit of a 'physiological explanation.' When irremedial bodily peculiarities are integrated with the whole of our experience, they cease to have the dignity of a cause in us. A visual anomaly can receive a universal signification by the mediation of the artist and become for him the occasion of perceiving one of the 'profiles' of human existence". (p. 203) A similar comment on Cézanne, "Heredity may well have given him rich sensations, strong emotions, and a vague feeling of anguish or mystery which upset the life he might have wished for himself and which cut him off from humanity; but these qualities cannot create a work of art without the expressive act, and they have no bearing on the difficulties or the virtues of that act." (1964, p. 69).

[11] "Visual contents are taken up, utilized and sublimated to the level of thought by a symbolical power which transcends them, but it is on the basis of sight that this power can be constituted. The relationship between matter and form is called in phenomenological terminology a relationship of *Fundeirung:* the symbolic function rests on the visual as on a ground: not that vision is its cause, but because it is that gift of nature which Mind was called upon to make use of [...]" (1945/1962, p. 127).

> and at others moves towards personal acts. Psychological motives and bodily occasions may overlap because there is not a single impulse in a living body which is entirely fortuitous in relation to psychic intentions, and not a single mental act which has not found at least its germ or its general outline in physiological tendencies (1945/1962, p. 88).

That which we traditionally call "mind", comprised of the cognitive processes associated with conscious thought, is just one level of mind. For example, my eyes focus upon a scene which I wish to see, and it becomes foreground and everything else fades into the background. This task is not accomplished by means of reflection or cognition, nor is it the result of causal processes. It is done as soon as *I wish* to see something. We need our eyes to see, but we don't see with our eyes, we see with sight. Sight is a lived relation between the lived body and the world. Merleau Ponty writes, "The eye is not the mind, but a material organ. How could it ever take anything 'into account'? It can only do so if we introduce the phenomenal body besides the objective one, if we make a knowing body of it, and if, in short, we substitute for consciousness, as the subject of perception, existence, or being in the world through a body." (1945/1962, p. 309, footnote). In this very basic perceptual way, the body is already an instrument of comprehension. Neither the eye as retinal structure nor thought as cognitive processes is responsible for being able to *look* at something. The "look" is to orient oneself in the display of the world, and this task is performed instantaneously, in the lived body (i.e. mind–body–world system). There is no mystery in this, but we need a phenomenological attitude in order to understand it, and a non-dualistic way of describing it.

Psychological motivations and bodily activity are woven together in the lived experience of existing in the world. The body is not an inert mass or thing which we must orchestrate into action, but rather the "living envelope" of all our intentions. We are an incarnated subject, living in concrete situations. The next step in this introduction to Merleau-Ponty's thought will be to examine the nature of the "dialogue" between the incarnate subject and the world. In this chapter we will only examine the early Merleau-Ponty, from the point of view of the lived body. In Chap. 4 we will see how he revises his concept of the lived body into the concept of the flesh.

The phenomenon of perception (our attending to the world through the body) is the place of interaction between the subject and its world. Our perceptual experience of the world is the only way in which we have access to that which is outside of ourselves. Merleau-Ponty's insight was to place perception at the center of the mystery of human existence. Perception "[…] is not a science of the world, it is not even an act, a deliberate taking up of a position; it is the background from which all acts stand out, and is presupposed by them. The world is not an object such that I have in my possession the law of its making: it is the natural setting of, and field for, all my thoughts and all my explicit perceptions." (1945/1962, 10–11). Perception brings together duration (existence as temporal), the unity of the world (the inter-subjective social world which we experience as the *same* for all) and the coherence of past and present (the historical, cultural world). In the early essay "The primacy of perception" (1964) he wrote: "By these words, the "primacy of perception" we mean that the experience of perception is our presence at the moment when things, truths, values are constituted for us [...]" (p. 25) and from the same text, "Should we now generalize and say that what is true of perception is also true in the order of the intellect and that in a general way all our experience, all our knowledge, has the same fundamental structures, the same synthesis of transition, the same kinds of horizons which we have found in perceptual experience?" (p. 19). Put another way, perception is the opening up of the body onto being. Merleau-Ponty's analysis of perception is an immense topic, but for the sake of focus and relevance for psychosomatics, I will here only highlight the way in which the body is involved in "meaning constitution", since the problematic of psychosomatics is precisely the anomaly of a "speaking body".

The lived body is to be understood as someone's lived relationship to the world. It is an ambiguous unity, both subject and object, both mind and body, intertwined, understood in terms of levels, or planes of signification rather than mutually exclusive categories of being.[12] Merleau-Ponty makes some distinctions in this unity, which will be helpful in understanding the anomaly of a "thinking" body. At the most fundamental level, Merleau-Ponty speaks of an anonymous, pre-personal bodily existence (*le moi naturel).*[13] Here we find a dimension of meaning at the body level, which is meaningful and intentional, although it is a lived meaning which is not thematic nor articulated at the order of reflective thoughts. This lived, body "meaning" provides us with stable, habitual functioning which is the general outline of that which gets taken up and transformed into the realm of the personal, psychological cultural level of existence. What is this level of meaning? For example, take the everyday experience of moving about in one's home. My body knows its way around my apartment, in what could be called knowledge of the legs.[14] Merleau-Ponty gives the example in *Phenomenology of Perception* of the woman who has a feather on her hat which she manages to keep at a distance from her surroundings so that it doesn't break off. She doesn't calculate this distance. She has incorporated the feather into her body. This kind of body knowledge is our bodily understanding of the world, a kind of harmony between that which we aim for (to get to the kitchen) and that which is given (the particular layout of the apartment). This level of meaning is neither to be understood as a mental content nor a stimuli-bound reflex. As body knowledge (when it becomes sedimented as habit), it is neither thematic knowledge nor involuntary

---

[12] Descartes usually gets blamed for the dualistic conceptualization of man in his famous divide between *Res extensa* and *Res cogitans,* resulting in the influential definition of man as "the thinking reed/thing".

[13] All perception takes place in an atmosphere of generality and is given to us as anonymous. I cannot say *I* see the blue of the sky in the sense in which I say I understand a book, or again in which I say I decide to devote my life to mathematics [...] if I want to render precisely the perceptual experience, I ought to say that *one* perceives in me, not that I perceive. (1945/1962, p. 215).

[14] "My flat is, for me, not a set of closely associated images. It remains a familiar domain round about me only as long as I still have "in my hands" or "in my legs" the main distances and directions involved, as long as from my body intentional threats run out towards it". (ibid, p. 130).

action. Merleau-Ponty calls this level of understanding for a pre-reflected “operative intentionality”, or “motor intentionality”.[15] This basic orientation in the world is the background which is sustains the meaning of movement, gives movement its’ very pre-condition as a possible projection into a meaningful world.[16] He uses a similar idea for this function on a psycho-social level, called “the intentional arc”, which gives us our world as already “there” as the implicit setting of one’s movements thoughts and actions. It is a form of life which places us in a situation which we already understand, beyond or below conscious awareness and thought. He describes the intentional arc in the following way:

> Beneath intelligence as beneath perception, we discover a more fundamental function [...] [which] makes objects exist in a more intimate sense for us. Let us therefore say rather [...] that the life of consciousness – cognitive life -, the life of desire or perceptual life – is subtended by an ‘intentional arc’ which projects round about us our past, our future, our human setting [...] which results in our being situated in all these respects. It is this intentional arc which brings about the unity of the senses, of intelligence, of sensibility and motility (1945/1962, pp. 135–136).

So we find in Merleau-Ponty a description of meaning which is not reserved for cognitive thought, a meaning that is a quiet constant constitution which is the pre-condition for having a human world.[17] My body already “has” the world in a primordial way. Another term Merleau-Ponty uses to explicate this level of meaning is body schema (*schéma corporel).* This term is not to be understood as psychologists use the term, but rather as a description of the intuitive understanding of one’s own the body and its position in space. One’s own body is the third term, always tacitly understood in the figure/ground structure. If the telephone is to the left of my desk, it is because I am to the right of the telephone. The body is not *in* space, it “inhabits” space. It is “[...] polarized by its tasks, of its *existence towards* them, of its collecting together of itself in its pursuits of its aim, the body image is finally a way of stating that my body is in the world.” (1945/1962, p. 101). There is always a setting in perception which pre-supposes this fundamental being situated.[18] This understanding is immediate and intuitive, never reflected upon. Merleau-Ponty illustrates this fundamental “being situated” by the

---

[15] Other thinkers have further developed this terminology, see Gallagher (1995) on “pre-noetic work” or Seamon’s (2000) “pre-cognitive intelligence of the body.”

[16] “It is not easy to reveal pure motor intentionality: it is concealed behind the objective world which it helps to build up. (1945/1962, p. 138 footnote).

[17] The word *sens* in French has a variety of meanings lacking in the English “meaning/signification”. *Sens* can mean: sensation, skill, intelligibility or direction. Meaning is thus connected to the body in its sensations, abilities and mobility, reiterating the intertwining of body, meaning and being-in-the-world. Merleau-Ponty uses the term *Être au monde* for being-in-the-world, which translates literally into being *towards* the world, again drawing attention to bodily tasks and engagements rather than being “in” the world, as being placed in a container.

[18] “Space is not the setting (real or logical) in which things are arranged, but the means whereby the position of things becomes possible” (1945/1962, p. 243).

term "habit", which has a special significance in this thinking.[19] Some quotes below on this:

> The acquisition of habit is indeed the grasping of a significance, but it is the motor grasping of a motor significance. Now what precisely does this mean? A woman may, without any calculation, keep a safe distance between the feather in her hat and the things that might break it off. She feels where the feather is just as we feel where our hand is. If I am in the habit of driving a car, I enter a narrow opening and see that I can "get through" without comparing the width of the opening with the width of the wings, just as I go through a doorway without checking the width of the doorway against that of my body. [...] To get used to a hat [or] a car [...] is to be transplanted into them, or conversely, to incorporate them into the bulk of our own body (1945/1962, p. 143).
>
> Habit expresses our power of dilating our being-in-the-world, or changing our existence by appropriating fresh instruments [...] To know how to type is not, then, to know the place of each letter among the keys [...] It is a knowledge in the hands, which is forthcoming only when bodily effort is made, and cannot be formulated in detachment from that effort (ibid, 143–144).
>
> But this power of habit is no different from the general one which we exercise over our body: if I am ordered to touch my ear or my knee, I move my hand to my ear or my knee by the shortest route, without having to think of the initial position of my hand, or that of my ear, or the path between them. We said earlier that it is the body which "understands" in the acquisition of habit [...] But the phenomenon of habit is just what prompts us to revise our notion of "understand" and our notion of the body. To understand is to experience the harmony between what we aim at what is given, between the intention and the performance – and our body is our anchorage in a world. When I put my hand to my knee, I experience as every stage of movement the fulfillment of an intention, which was not directed at my knee as an idea or even as an object, but as a present and real part of my living body, that is, finally as a stage in my perpetual movement towards a world. When the typist performs the necessary movements on the typewriter, these movements are governed by an intention, but the intention does not posit the keys as objective locations. It is literally true that the subject who learns to type incorporates the key-bank space into his bodily space (ibid, p. 144).

The "meaning" explicated in the phenomenon of habit reveals an intentionality that is both bodily and existential, which means that intentionality is not a matter of consciousness flashing a flashlight on various areas objects arrayed before it (remnants of the idealism Merleau-Ponty disliked in Husserl's phenomenology), but the constitution of an embodied subject and world simultaneously. Meaning is that which emerges from the concrete encounter between the world that shows itself (affords itself) in relation to those tasks, interests and attentions that the subject brings to the scene. Meaning is virtual for Merleau-Ponty, not real, like a thing, nor ideal, like a thought. It emerges as the world and the subject carve our each other "somewhere in the middle." This intertwining, taking place on all levels, is a direct challenge to traditional ontology (subject—object dichotomy) and the natural attitude way of thinking.[20] It defies the objectivistic epistemology

---

[19] Dreyfus (1996) points out that when uses the word "habit" he often means skill, that is, to be able to *do*.

[20] "In short, my body is not only an object among all other objects, a nexus of sensible qualities among others, but an object which is *sensitive to* all the rest, which reverberates to all sounds,

(the God's eye view) and places the body into philosophy in a fundamental way. He does not place one "sector of the field" (mind–body–world) as first or primordial, although he does in his early work use Husserl's notion of *fundiering* (founded upon) to describe the relationship between the anonymous, body level and the personal, psychological, cultural level. Not only are the higher levels founded on the lower, Merleau-Ponty means that much of our existence is played out on this lower, pre-reflected level of habit. The phenomenon of habit allows Merleau-Ponty to develop an important concept for his phenomenology of the lived body, namely the notion of "structure" and structure transformation. I will be using Merleau-Ponty's notion of structure and structure transformation in my psychosomatic theory developed in Chap. 5, so let me end this chapter by presenting Merleau-Ponty's concepts of "structure" and "structure transformation", which will be an important part of understanding psychosomatic pathology."

Structure and Structure Transformation

Merleau-Ponty's notion of structure was first presented in *The Structure of Behavior* from 1942, where his primary aim was to criticize the causal, mechanical thinking which had infiltrated philosophy and psychology. He considered the Gestalt psychologists' notion of "form" to be a step in the right direction, but not radical enough. His use of the term "structure" was his improvement on the concept of form, freed from Gestalt psychology's naturalistic bias. Structures are not really out there in the world (the naturalistic fallacy he accused Gestalt psychologists of making), nor completely constituted by consciousness. They are rather the result of the meeting of the two, a familiar theme by now. Structures are the meaningful signification of the lived. Structures are the bodily, psychological, socio-cultural patterns which lead us in our experience of the world, but they are also formed by our encounter with the world. Once again, we find the metaphor of dialogue to describe the meeting between man and the world. Structures are our attunement to the world, on all levels, whereby we take in "something" which is other than ourselves, get a "grip" on this "something" (be it bodily or at the level of mind) and when understanding occurs, a kind of "harmony" with that which presents itself is achieved. We gradually integrate this experience as a habitual way of relating to and understanding the world. Thus, our experiences are a constant flux of encounters with the familiar (using habitual sedimented structures) as well as encounters with the new and unfamiliar, which create a tension or disharmony, requiring a transformation of habitual structures in order to accommodate the new. When structures are transformed and sedimented, they become a

(Footnote 20 continued)
vibrates to all colors, and provides words with their primordial significance through the way in which it receives them." (1945/1962, p. 236).

part of our habitual way of being in the world, thus expanding and further articulating our experiences. The dialogue between man and world is an ever on-going process. The world continually presents us with a rudimentary organization, unfinished and beckoning, which calls for our participation or response.

Being at grips with the world means having structures with which one can meaningfully experience the world. These structures, once in place, cannot be nullified. However, since the world is inexhaustible, in that it is always beyond the given, like a horizon, ever changing and transforming, I am constantly challenged to be prepared to transform my habitual (sedimented) structures. The more I deepen and articulate my understanding of the world, the more of the world is shown to me. This is the human condition, to be an embodied subject, already in the world that is familiar on a deep level (motor intentionality and intentional arc), yet constantly being challenged to modify and overturn sedimented "ready- made" significations when necessary. Thus, two major characteristics of structures are that they are sedimented into habitual patterns but also "spontaneous", that is to say, capable of transformation.

To illustrate this rather difficult notion of structures, let me take some examples from *The Structure of Behavior*. Here, Merleau-Ponty gives some examples from the animal world. At the lowest level of animal existence, we find the simple reflex response.[21] Higher up, there are animals who can respond to a variety of situations which could not be handled by reflex behavior. These animals respond to a type of *configuration*, a level of reality which has been disengaged from material properties. It is this openness or ambiguity in the perception of this situation which allows for a certain degree of flexibility on the animal's response. A monkey can learn to pick "the lighter color" or is able to understand that the chocolate is always under "the last box" and so on. Thus, the higher animals can understand the *form or structure* of the situation. They have succeeded in discerning the structure of signals from their material properties (not this or that particular box, but the box which happens to be the *last one*). The more complex the configurations are, and the higher the degree of freedom in the animal's response, the more "intelligent" we call the behavior. In the same work, Merleau-Ponty recounts an interesting experiment where fish that had learned to eat both white bread and black bread were fed white chalk mixed together with the white bread. It was observed that the fish could only very slowly and arduously learn to ignore the chalk and eat only the white bread. What was interesting was that when these same fish were then fed black bread mixed together with pieces of black rubber, they learned very quickly to ignore the rubber. Merleau-Ponty comments, "It is not to a certain material that

---

[21] Even simple reflex behavior is critically examined by Merleau-Ponty in *The Structure of Behavior*, where he demonstrates that even these seemingly automatic behaviors are never completely indifferent to both the internal and external situation. The rhythm and location of the stimulus, for example, will determine whether or not the reflex is released. The classical account of reflex as blind automatic is thus called into question, in favor of understanding reflexes as behavior which tends to balance itself in accordance with preferred patterns of distribution. See pp. 10–33.

the animal has adapted, but to speak a human language, to a certain kind of deception [...] It is an aptitude of choosing, or a 'method of selection' which is established (1942/1963, p. 97). In other words, a very rudimentary structure had become sedimented for the fish, and as structure they were able to apply the lesson from the initial situation with the white bread to a similar one with the black bread. The structure "some particles which look like food are in fact not food" had found its way into the world of the fish. Animals may discern a structure, but only man can *create* a structure. Experiments have shown that a chimpanzee can understand to use a box to stand on the reach something, but will not use the same box as a seat. The thing remains only a "box to stand on". In other words, the chimpanzee was not capable of assuming a *point of view* in relation to the box. They could not freely choose which aspect of the thing would emerge in a particular field, or situation.[22] Man is the only animal who has a point of view, who can transform the significance of the scene, who can have a *possible world.*

Structures are the bodily, psychological and social ways of being oriented towards the world that guide our understanding and through sedimentation give us freedom by presenting the world as familiar and known. Our habitual, sedimented structures allow us to experience the world as comprehensible and manageable. We develop stable patterns of experience that tell us how to move our bodies, how to respond to various psychological and social situations, and how to understand our everyday ordinary life-world. These structures, built up over time, free our attention from having to form the "base" of experience over and over again. Our maternal language and bodily repertoire are second nature to us. We do not have to re-learn them in every new situation. Such sedimentations are the necessary pre-condition for us to be able to communicate fluently and move about in an unencumbered way. The experience of learning a new language or a new motor skill makes us aware of how effortlessly these sedimented structures actually work. To have to think about which verb form to use or where to put the negation in a sentence shows us what language is like when it is *not* part of a sedimented structure. However, if we learn the new language well enough and use it for a long enough time, we may reach the point where even the second language becomes a part of our sedimented language repertoire. In such a case, we have expanded our language structure. The ability to learn a new language is an example of how structures are not only sedimented but also spontaneous. This means that we can develop our structures to fit new situations and challenges.

The way in which structures are formed, change and develop can be illustrated by the experience of learning to drive a car. Before one can drive, the car is experienced merely as a means of transportation, or perhaps as a source of aesthetic pleasure. The "car-structure" is not articulated in a nuanced way, but generalized, with little detail. Perceptually, I attend to the car door, the seat, perhaps the smell of the car and the sound of the engine, but over and above these blunt impressions nothing particular stands out. In terms of motility, the car-structure of the

---

22 This example is also from *The Structure of Behavior.*

non-driver has to do with the way one moves one's body into get to the car, the feeling of the seat (on the passenger side), the passing view from the window. Before one can drive, the experience of the car will be at this level of articulation. However, all of this changes as soon as I place myself in the driver's seat and start to learn to drive. Firstly, my body will no longer be passively "seated" in the car seat, but must become actively attuned to the pedals, stick shift, mirrors and steering wheel. The view from the window that was so entertaining and free from demands as a passenger suddenly becomes filled with questions (Which lane should I be in? When should I signal? Should I pass this car?) and demands (he is waiting for me to turn? I seem to be blocking traffic, I just missed a chance to enter the roundabout, they keep passing me, I'm probably driving too slowly, everyone is honking at me). When I listen to the engine as the driver, the sound is no longer experienced as the background noise of "starting the car" but rather a noise to be queried: how does the engine sound? Is everything all right? In the first phases of learning to drive, I will have to filter every perception and motor activity through cognition, as there is as yet no sedimented structure for this experience. I will be hyper-present to my own body, to the various instruments of the car and to the traffic in a way that experienced drivers have long forgotten. The passage from novice to experienced driver is accomplished when I "have" the road and the car in my body. The driving becomes a harmonious field of experience where I move with ease. I am no longer hyper-aware of myself driving, nor am I in need of constant cognition in order to navigate the car in traffic. I can even lose myself in thought and not realize how I suddenly arrived at home. There have even been reported incidences of people driving in their sleep as a side-effect of a certain type of sleeping medication. To an inexperienced driver, this sounds like an impossible feat.

Merleau-Ponty's notion of the lived body and structure transformation provides a philosophical alternative to the objectivistic epistemology that focuses on the objective body, as seen from a God's eye perspective. The lived body is understood as a mind-body presence always directed towards the world (otherness). Therein a field arises, an "in-between", that is constituted in terms of situations to be mastered and understood. The term "meaning" is expanded in Merleau-Ponty's work, through the introduction of the concepts body schema, motor intentionality, intentional arc, habit-body, structure and structure transformation. Studying the phenomenon of perception phenomenologically gives us access to a previously unexplored territory, which Merleau-Ponty describes in various ways as the intertwining or "dialogue" between man and world. All these concepts are extremely fruitful in order to by-pass the unsolvable mysteries surrounding psychosomatics. In the following chapter we will take a closer look at "meaning" in order to prepare the ground for a new understanding of psychosomatics in terms of the lived body.

References

Bredlau, S. M. (2011). A respectful world: Merleau-Ponty and the experience of depth. *Human Studies, 33*, 411–423.

Brentano, F. (1982). *Descriptive psychology*. Hamburg: Felix Meiner Verlag.

Carman, T. (2008). *Merleau-Ponty*. London: Routledge.

Diprose, R., & Reynolds, J. (Eds.). (2008). *Merleau-Ponty: Key concepts*. Stocksfield: Acumen Press.

Dreyfus, H. (1996). The current relevance of Merleau-Ponty's phenomenology of embodiment. *The Electronic Journal of Analytic philosophy, 4*(spring issue), 1–16. doi: 10.1145/1690388.1690464.

Hass, L. (2008). *Merleau-Ponty's philosophy*. Bloomington: Indiana University Press.

Husserl, E. (1913/1962). *Ideas: General introduction to pure phenomenology* (Vol. 1). New York: Collier Books.

Husserl, E. (1954/1970). *Crisis of European sciences and transcendental phenomenology*. Evanston: Northwestern University Press.

Merleau-Ponty, M. (1942/1963). *The structure of behavior*. Boston: Beacon Press.

Merleau-Ponty, M. (1945/1962). *Phenomenology of perception*. London: Routledge & Kegan Paul.

Merleau-Ponty, M. (1948/1964). *Sense and non-sense*. Evanston Illinois: Northwestern University Press.

Merleau-Ponty, M. (1960/1964). *Signs*. Evanston Illinois: Northwestern University Press.

Merleau-Ponty, M. (1964a). The primacy of perception. In J. M. Edie (Ed.), *The primacy of perception: And other essays on phenomenological psychology, the philosophy of art, history and politics* (pp. 12–42). Evanston Illinois: Northwestern University Press.

Merleau-Ponty, M. (1964/1973). *Consciousness and the acquisition of language*. Evanston Illinois: Northwestern University Press.

Merleau-Ponty, M. (1964/1968). *The visible and the invisible*. Evanston Illinois: Northwestern University Press.

Merleau-Ponty, M. (1969/1973). *The Prose of the world*. Evanston Illinois: Northwestern University Press.

Nagel, T. (1989). *The view from nowhere*. New York: Oxford University Press.

Seamon, D. (2000). *A way of seeing people and place: Phenomenology in environment-behavior research*. New York: Klewer Academic/Plenum publishers.

Spiegelberg, H. (1982). *The phenomenological movement*. The Hague: Martinus Nijhoff Publishers.

Chapter 3
The Meaning of Meaning

In this chapter we will be looking at the notion of "meaning", an important concept for the understanding of psychosomatic pathology. As seen in Chap. 1, all traditional psychosomatic theories have included a meaning component in their etiological explanations of psychosomatic pathology, although none has given a satisfactory account of how meaning (the "psycho" in psychosomatic) is transformed into body. In the previous chapter, I have shown that Merleau-Ponty's phenomenological concept of the lived body provides an alternative way of conceptualizing mind, body and world as well as a description of how mind, body and world "work together" in order to enable the experience of the human world. In this chapter, I will through Merleau-Ponty's expanded notion of meaning, illustrate how his philosophy once again provides a fruitful alternative to classical thinking, an alternative which we need in order to properly understand psychosomatics.[1]

The concept of "meaning" traditionally has to do with language, specifically the relationship of language to that which is referred to in the world, that is, the connection between the word and its so-called designated object. A linguistic statement is said to have meaning (makes sense) if it is comprehensible, in terms of content (semantics) and syntax for a native speaker. A statement does not need to be true, in the sense of corresponding to actual states of affairs in the world, in order to be meaningful, but it must be comprehensible. Noam Chomsky once coined the famous sentence "colorless green ideas sleep furiously" in order to show that although a sentence may be grammatically correct, it may nevertheless be semantically incomprehensible. Conversely, we may have sentences with unusual syntax, as in poetry, but still find them semantically meaningful. Modern philosophical work on meaning treats the subject in terms of how people communicate (so-called audience directed intentions of speakers/speech acts), what conditions must be met in order for language to be able to make truthful statements

[1] I will not be going into all the finer points of his thinking on language, as it would take us to far from the focus of this book, which is an application of some Merleau-Pontian philosophy on the phenomenon of psychosomatics.

J. Bullington, *The Expression of the Psychosomatic Body from a Phenomenological Perspective*, SpringerBriefs in Philosophy,
DOI: 10.1007/978-94-007-6498-9_3, © The Author(s) 2013

about the world, and matters of interpretation and translation.[2] We will not be going into these debates as they are not specifically relevant to the aim of this chapter. Language and meaning will be discussed here as expressions of a particular human way of being—in- the- world. This phenomenological perspective on meaning will be useful in order to understand the formation of psychosomatic symptoms explicated in Chap. 5.

Without a doubt, human beings live in a world formed by language. We are the kind of creatures we are because of our ability to use language in a symbolic way. The philosopher Cassirer (1944) pointed out in his early essay on language in *Essay on Man,* that only humans can be said to possess the language *function.* Many higher animals can use signs to designate wants or desires in various situations, but only human beings can use language freed from the concrete here- and-now situation. A chimp can learn to point at a card with a banana on it when it is hungry, or can even be taught to construct simple sentences, but only when motivated by need (hunger) or reward (experimental situations). The use of signs by animals remains stimuli- bound and non-creative. Only the human can think about bananas when s/he is not hungry, paint a banana, write a poem or a song about a banana (the so-called "displaced reference") and so on. Humans think abstractly and symbolically, subsume objects under categories, apply logical thinking (either/or, negation, causality etc.), develop syntax, create temporal distinctions in verb forms, make use of metaphors and metonymy, lie and fantasize, make jokes and understand irony. None of this is possible without the language function. The origin and development of human language is an intriguing question. When did *homo sapiens* start to speak in a human way? Cave carvings from 70,000 years ago found in Africa would suggest that these ancient relatives had the capacity for symbolic thought. How did such a thing come about?

The anthropologist Maxine Sheets-Johnstone (1990) criticizes the traditional view that increased brains size or hunting behavior was responsible for the origin of human language, in favor of what she calls a sensory—kinetic model. She concedes that brain size and various behaviors can account for the *beginning* of language, but not its *origin.* Sheets-Johnstone's theory is that the possibility for verbal language resides in the oral anatomy of the human tongue.[3] The infant's exploration of the mother's nipple in breast feeding provides the first tactile experiences of the tongue (as touch*ing*, not just as touched). This initial oral exploration of the world on the part of the infant has been pointed out by both Freud and Piaget. Sheets-Johnstone adds that it is actually the *motility* of the tongue (as opposed to the fixated position

[2] See Taylor (1985) for an introduction to meaning theory. Other writers of interest in this area are Davidson, D., Dennet, D., Dummet, M., Fodor, J., Grice, H.P., Strawson, P.F., Quine, W., Wittgenstein, L.

[3] Other scholars have pointed out that bipedality changed the position of the skull, allowing for the larynx to make specifically human sounds, especially the vowels. On a social level, it has been hypothesized that as soon as man started to use more tools, his hands were occupied and could no longer gesture with his hands. For that reason, making sounds replaced making motor gestures in order to communicate. Communication in the dark would also be a situation requiring sound.

of the lips) which allows the tongue to act like a small finger, investigating by touch the physiognomy of objects, as smooth, hard, warm, cold, flat, round, beginning and end, dry or moist etc. Verbal identification of objects presupposes the initial differentiation of things according to how they qualitatively appear. According the Sheets-Johnstone, this first differentiation is performed by the tongue. In this experience we find the first introduction to a world of distinctions. The tongue is the first animate organ, the first sensory-kinetic power in relation to a qualitatively distinct world. Later on, the infant plays with sounds. Thanks to the movement of the tongue, different ranges of sounds can be made. In babbling, the infant discovers the tongue is a source of sound, as well as a touching instrument. The baby makes sounds which attract the attention of the parents, and through imitation, s/he approximates the same kinds of sounds as they make, the closer the imitation, the greater the enthusiasm from the parents. Thus, babbling allows the infant to discover how to make sounds that elicit a positive response, resulting in the infants' internalization of the phonetic sounds of the native language. So, before there can be verbal language, there must be an awareness of oneself as the sound-maker. Sheets-Johnstone reasons that what is a necessary pre-condition for verbal language in the infant must have also been necessary for the first *homo sapiens* who spoke. They may not have babbled like the infant, but they must have made the discovery that they could make sounds and differentiate between them. After these preconditions are met, the coupling together of sounds and concrete situations, such as danger, food, sexual excitement, emotional exclamations and so on, developed into a gestural level of language, much like the sign level of language described above with animals, tied to concrete here- and- now situations. How this primitive gestural language then developed into symbolic language is a debated issue. Was it due to an innate capacity found in the brain, so-called "innate structures"? Was it a mutation, resulting in instantaneously language capacity that then survived because of its evolutionary benefits? Or did language gradually evolve from social interaction? From song? It is generally regarded as difficult to answer this question since it happened so far back in time. Finding tools at archeological digs can give evidence that language was in use, since the inhabitants would have had to be able to give instructions on how to build and use the tools, but exactly how and why language developed is impossible to say.

The mystery of human language is that we understand what it means to "mean" something. I may point my finger to show my cat a mouse or a bird, but he will look only at my finger, not at what I am pointing at. He doesn't understand what it means to point. However, he does understand quite a bit about the world. He looks at the door when he wants to go out, stands by his bowl when he wants food. But the step from this level of understanding of the world to the human world of language is immense. Although we cannot say how this evolutionary step came about, the way in which we live the world as articulated by meaning and language is one of the "givens" in human experience. Let us now turn to see how Merleau-Ponty widens the concept of meaning so that it can be understood as an "in-between" phenomena (in-between mind and body and in-between mind/body and world), giving us a way to leave behind the unfruitful dichotomies of ordinary thinking.

Merleau-Ponty on Meaning and Expression

In *Phenomenology of Perception* (especially the chapter "The body as expression, and speech") Merleau-Ponty presents his early thoughts on language. Here, Merleau-Ponty argues against the view that words and speech are simply a way of designating thoughts and things in favor of understanding language as the very *presence* of thought and things for the human being in the world. Thoughts and things (as designated/named objects) are not external to my perception and experience of them, rather, they are *formed by* this experience and perception. The speaker does not translate ready-made thoughts in his head into spoken language. It is by the act of speaking that the human world is accomplished. We live in a world where speech is already inscribed, as an institution, in our way of being and we are not surprised by the inter-subjective world, we take it for granted as *the world.* "[...] it is within a world already spoken and speaking that we think." (1945/1962, p. 184). Language is a certain "style" of being-with-the world. But what can be said about of the origin of this way of being? How to "[...] find beneath the chatter of words, the primordial silence [...] and describe the action which breaks this silence." (ibid, 184).

In his early work, Merleau-Ponty writes that the meaning of words must be formed through a deduction from what he calls a "gestural language". The spoken word is described as a gesture, the meaning of which is to give us a world. Gestures are immediately understood. A gesture is a bodily expression that is one with its meaning. The gesture of shaking one's fist in anger and its meaning (an expression of anger) are one. In the same way that I perceive things with my body, I understand other people's gestures, with an immediacy that needs no intervening cognitions. We can imagine that this form of meaning was surely available to the first *homo sapiens*. But Merleau-Ponty is aware that a gestural theory of meaning is not the whole answer, for he asks, how did the available meanings themselves come to be constituted? There is also the problem of the arbitrariness of the word (sign) and the signified which brings language further from the intrinsic (often emotional) meaning of the gesture. Traditionally, it is said that a gesture is a "natural sign" and the word a "natural convention". Gesture aims at the sensible world of actions (perception, body and emotion) while speech aims at an already constituted, sedimented system of meanings (conditioned by language and culture). How do you get from gesture to cultural meaning? According to Barbaras (2004) Merleau-Ponty is still stuck in his affinity for naturalism and Gestalt psychology in his early writings, and therefore unable to get past the nature—culture dichotomy, which means that the duality between subject and object merely reappears in the form of an opposition between the natural world and the cultural world. He does not yet, according to Barbaras, grasp speech as an originary phenomenon, as he will do later on. Merleau-Ponty attempts to dissolve this dichotomy metaphorically in *Phenomenology of Perception*, that is, we can understand speech as a *kind of gesture*, but we still do not understand how a gesture can "speak", which is again, the problem of the *origin* of language.

Merleau-Ponty will pay a great deal of attention to this issue in his writings after *Phenomenology of Perception.*

What does language actually express? Not thoughts, according to Merleau-Ponty, but rather, the subject takes up of a position in the world of his meanings, which he "has" in the same way he already has his own body.

> The identity of the thing through perception experience is only another aspect of the identity of one's own body throughout exploratory movements; thus they are the same in kind as each other. Like the body image, the fireplace is a system of equivalents not founded on the recognition of some law, but on the experience of bodily presence. I become involved in things with my body, they co-exist with me as an incarnate subject, and this life among things has nothing in common with the elaboration of scientifically conceived objects. In the same way, I do not understand the gestures of others by some act of intellectual interpretation [...] The act by which I lend myself to the spectacle must be recognized as irreducible to anything else. I join it in a kind of blind recognition which precedes the intellectual working out and clarification of the meaning (1945/1962, p. 185).

What can be said about the actual acquisition of meaning and the spontaneous creation of new meaning? Merleau-Ponty explains this ability existentially, as a part of human nature that can appropriate significant cores or gestalts which transcend the current situation. This is first seen in terms of acquiring a new pattern of behavior (a capacity we share with the higher animals), then in the mute communication of gestures (infants and primitive man) and finally at the psychosocial level (involving spoken language and sedimented cultural meanings). It is the same "power" that allows the body to open up to a new kind of behavior that allows for the inception of the signification of sounds (as words). This is not miraculous, according to Merleau-Ponty, but just as natural as the emergence of gesture from the un-coordinated movements of the infant. In his early work, Merleau-Ponty calls this capacity man's inherent drive towards transcendence, this continual surpassing of the current state of affairs. The apprehension of a signification (meaning) is the opening up of a new horizon, which has both bodily and mental layers. Just as the act of my body has a certain hold on the world that makes it meaningful to me, so does the lived act of speech have a certain hold on a field of significations that organizes them in a useful and meaningful way. The ability of language to pull significations together is compared to the human body's ability to organize the perceptual field.

In an attempt to bridge perception and the psychosocial level of meaning, Merleau-Ponty writes in *Phenomenology of Perception* that instead of vacillating between "motility" and "intelligence" and wondering how they relate to each other, we need a third notion in order to integrate them, a function that operates at all levels, supporting the edifice of language, which is nevertheless relatively autonomous. He uses the example of the brain damaged patient Schneider to exemplify this function, by showing how it is missing in Schneider. Schneider speaks rarely and nearly only when he questioned, or if he himself asks a question it is a stereotyped phrase, always spoken in the same way. He never uses language to create a *possible situation*. He can only speak when he has prepared his sentences. He has no loss of intellect due to his injury, but he never feels like speaking.

His speech is ossified, as Merleau-Ponty puts it. The intention to speak requires openness to a horizon of possible meanings, a creativity and productivity, which Schneider lacks. Normal speech is constantly productive and transcending, a moving, ever opening-up upon the possible: "This ever-recreated opening in the plenitude of being is what conditions the child's first use of speech and the language of the writer, as it does the construction of the word and that of concepts. Such is the function which we intuit through language, which reiterates itself, which is its own foundation, or which, like a wave, gathers and poises itself to hurl beyond its own limits." (1945/1962, p. 197). The spontaneous creation of meaning is an example of this transcendence, which is characteristic of human beings.

The concept of meaning, described in this way, is understood as an existential capacity of the human being towards transcendence, taking behavioral or psycho-social form. Language is a specifically human way of being-in-the-world, a way of a way of reaching through space to be "with" the thing. According to Merleau-Ponty, the capacity of the body to take up new behaviors is an example of the same, anonymous power that allows for the origin and evolution of language. The primordial, gestural expression of the body is then refined and developed through language and culture, gradually resulting in an articulated human world. This is as far as Merleau-Ponty gets in *Phenomenology of Perception.* Let me now move on to some later works,[4] to further explicate the meaning of meaning in Merleau-Ponty's thought, where he develops his notion of "expression".

The duality between perception and higher order levels of meaning was a problem Merleau-Ponty attempted to address in his writings after *Phenomenology of Perception.* The refinement of the concept of "expression" became the way to integrate motility and intelligence on a deeper level. By "expression" Merleau-Ponty means the spontaneous birth of the whole (the "event") which gives us perception, other selves, past present and future, the natural and cultural world, in one weave of the cloth, so to speak. In expression, there are no longer disparate elements to be somehow "put together", but an original upsurge that is the human being-in-the-world, a holistic "expressive field". In the development of his thought, Merleau-Ponty gradually moves from phenomenological intentionality (*noesis/ noema)* towards a circularity which will in his last work, *The Visible and the Invisible,*[5] become what he calls "philosophical interrogation". During the period leading up to this last work, Merleau-Ponty worked with the question of language and sense- making in order try to capture the unitary vision put forth in his notion of "expression." He imagined that the relationship between language and experience is circular in that language folds back on the sense world to help articulate it, but it is a linguistic structure itself that is called forth by perception. Thus, "sense making" is no longer something to be merely understood as an accomplishment on

---

[4] See especially *Signs* (1960/1964a, b), *The Prose of the World (*1969/1973), *Consciousness and the Acquisition of Language* (1964/1973).

[5] The first working titles of this book were *The Origin of Truth (L'Origine de la vérité), The Geneology of the True/Real (Généalogie du vrai), Being and world* (*Être et monde),* indicating the move from phenomenology to ontology.

the part of the subject (the subject intending its' object-as-meant, the dichotomy implicit in intentionality) but also the way in which the world "affords" us certain possible experiences through the sedimentation of our bodily and psycho-social structures. There is a fundamental ambiguity in expression, as we express ourselves through language, but language forms our expression.[6] Expression is not the work of consciousness but rather a unity of being that brings forth both human embodied consciousness and that which one is conscious of in one simultaneous event. We do not discover ourselves and then discover a world. We exist in the unity of a movement (expression) where world and man are born together, a movement which has been poorly understood until now.

> [...] the spirit of the world is ourselves as soon as we know how *to move ourselves* and *to look.* These simple acts already contain the secret of expressive action [...] I want to go over there, and here I am, without access to the inhuman secret of bodily mechanisms [...] I look where the goal is, I am drawn by it [...] My glance towards the goal already has its own miracles [...] It is not the object which draws movements of accommodation and convergence (from the eyes). On the contrary, it has been demonstrated that I would never see anything clearly and that there would be no object for me unless I used my eyes *in such a way* as to make the view of a single object possible [...] It is our glances themselves, their synergy, their exploration, and their prospecting which bring the immanent object into focus [...] We must therefore recognize that what we call a "glance" a "hand," and in general the "body" constitute a system of systems devoted to the inspection of the world and capable of leaping over distances, piercing the perceptual future, and outlines, in the inconceivable platitude of being, hollows and reliefs, distances and gaps – in short, a meaning (1969/1973, p. 77–78).

Thus, all perception is primordial expression, as the "[...] primary operation which first constitutes signs as signs, makes that which is expressed dwell in them through the eloquence of their arrangement and configuration alone, implants a meaning in that which did not have one, and thus – far from exhausting itself in the instant at which it occurs – inaugurates an order and founds an institution or a tradition." (ibid, p. 67) Expression is not derived from perception, but perception is possible because of human expression, the human way of being thrown into a natural and psychosocial world.

Language and Expression

What is the role of language in expression (that gives us simultaneously ourselves, each other and the world)?[7] Language is not merely one example among many that

[6] This ambiguity will be explicated in his notion of reversibility, from his last work *The Visible and the Invisible*.

[7] Merleau-Ponty had read Saussure, whose writings exerted an influence in *The Prose of the World,* which was to be his treatise on the philosophy of language. However, he seemed to have lost interest in this project after 1952, abandoning it entirely in 1959. The book has been published as a posthumous, unfinished work, and according to Claude Lefort's introduction, it is

constitute the human world, but in fact is the privileged mode of human understanding. Through understanding language, we discover the human world. We may think that we understand language, but the moment we begin to reflect on what language is, and what it accomplishes, we find it hard to understand how signs/ words can have such a power. Language gives us the world by being transparent itself, "In the way it works, language hides itself from us. Its triumph is to efface itself and take us beyond the words to the author's very thoughts, so that we imagine we are engaged with him in a wordless meeting of the minds. Once worlds have cooled and been reaffixed to the page as signs, their very power to project us far away from themselves makes it impossible for us to believe they are the source of so many thoughts". (Merleau-Ponty 1969/1973, p. 10). We would not be interested in reading books or listening to the talk of others if it only told us what we already know. By using familiar signs (words and syntax) language carries one into a new fresh way of looking at the world and strange new meanings can emerge. To illustrate the unitary nature of expression (how it not only unties the subject with the world of things but also to others), Merleau-Ponty writes that when speaking or listening, I project myself into the world of the other person. Language transports me into the other. It is the "reverberation of my relations with others (ibid, p. 20).

> When I am listening, it is not necessary that I have an *auditory perception* of the articulated sounds but that the conversation pronounces itself within me. It summons me and grips me; it envelopes and inhabits me to the point that I cannot tell what comes from me and what from it (ibid, p. 19).

The relationship between language and meaning is like the relationship between body and mind, the one is neither primary nor secondary to the other, they are intertwined levels of one expression "[...] language is not meaning's servant, and yet it does not govern meaning. There is no subordination between them. Here no one commands and no one obeys. What we *mean* is not before us, outside all speech, as sheer signification. It is only the excess of what we live over what has already been said. With our apparatus of expression we set ourselves up in a situation the apparatus is sensitive to, we confront it with the situation, and our statements are only the final balance of these exchanges." (1969/1973, p. 83). Meanings emerge from a context we are already familiar with (as sedimented reproduction of the known) but may take on a spontaneous new form in a dynamic process, accomplishing an opening up of new aspects of the world, on all levels of existence. This description is reminiscent of his characterization of structures in *Phenomenology of Perception,* which exhibit tendencies towards habituation (sedimentation) as well as the creative, spontaneous power of transformation (new behaviors and new meanings). In sum, the human capacity for language and thought are merely an extension of our embodied life, which includes the natural

---

(Footnote 7 continued)
not likely that Merleau-Ponty would have finished it if he had lived, at least not in the form we have today. I will not go into Saussure's influence on Merleau-Ponty's thought as it would stray too far from the focus of the chapter, for those interested see Hass (2008) and Barbaras (2004).

powers of sedimentation (habit formation) and transformation (creation of new meaning) on all levels, a power that enables a world to emerge as comprehensible and capable of developing into ever further levels of articulation.

The lesson we learn from Merleau-Ponty's notion of expression and his unitary vision of the birth of meaning as the meeting between the subject and the world is that we must put aside our natural attitude conceptions of "meaning" as cognitive content and see meaning in its more primordial role as the simultaneous articulation of world and subject. Meaning is the way in which the human beings' body and mind (higher levels of articulation through language and culture) are oriented towards a world which is also "in the making". As bodily and mental structures are formed and used to interpret the world, the world folds back upon these structures, constantly changing and readjusting them. This movement is often described in Merleau-Ponty's texts in terms of a "moving equilibrium". The subject and the world are always in the process of becoming. The subject acts in the world with needs, interests and desires and receives back from the world only from within the context of these needs, desires and interests. There is no inherent "meaning" in the world independent of the living, embodied subject involved in concrete situations. Thus, meaning is understood as the system of moving equilibrium that constantly goes from tension (in terms of unfilled intentions, ambiguity, new situations) to harmony (reaching the goal, finding the solution, sedimenting the new into the known) in a continuous flow of the "in-between" which is human experience of the world.

When "meaning" is thus freed from its connection to cognitive content, it is no longer problematic to conceive of a "speaking body" which has given psychosomatic theory so much trouble. But before we are ready for the re-interpretation of psychosomatics presented in Chap. 5, we need to follow Merleau-Ponty into his last work, *The Visible and the Invisible* where the unitary vision of the "event" of meaning will find its fulfillment in a new ontology, the ontology of the flesh.

References

Barbaras, R. (2004). *The being of the phenomenon*. Bloomington: Indiana University Press.

Cassirer, E. (1944). *An essay on man*. New Haven: Yale University Press.

Hass, L. (2008). *Merleau-Ponty's philosophy*. Bloomington: Indiana University Press.

Merleau-Ponty, M. (1945/1962). *Phenomenology of perception*. London: Routledge & Kegan Paul.

Merleau-Ponty, M. (1960/1964). *Signs*. Evanston Illinois: Northwestern University Press.

Merleau-Ponty, M. (1964/1973). *Consciousness and the acquisition of language*. Evanston Illinois: Northwestern University Press.

Merleau-Ponty, M. (1964/1968). *The visible and the invisible*. Evanston Illinois: Northwestern University Press.

Merleau-Ponty, M. (1969/1973). *The prose of the world*. Evanston Illinois: Northwestern University Press.

Sheets-Johnstone, M. (1990). *The roots of thinking*. Philadelphia: Temple University Press.

Taylor, C. (1985). *Theories of meaning in human Agency and language, Philosophical papers I*. Cambridge: Cambridge University press.

Chapter 4
The Lived Body (*Phenomenology of Perception*) and the Flesh (*The Visible and the Invisible*)

Most Merleau-Ponty scholars agree that Merleau-Ponty was not satisfied with his *Phenomenology of Perception* (1945/1962), fearing that the ambiguity he described in the notion of the lived body, as the intertwining of mind and body, subject and world, was a "bad ambiguity" that left behind insoluble problems.[1] He wrote in his working notes to *The Visible and the Invisible*[2]: "The problems posed in phenomenology of perception are insoluble because I start there from the 'consciousness' – 'object' distinction" (p. 200). He came to the conclusion that a strict adherence to the intentionality of consciousness leads to a "phenomenological positivism" that he must ultimately reject, "All consciousness is consciousness of something or of the world, but this *something*, this *world*, is no longer, as 'phenomenological positivism' appeared to teach, an object that is what it is, exactly adjusted to acts of consciousness" (1993, p. 70). Although there are germs of some of the ideas which Merleau-Ponty will develop in *The Visible and the Invisible* already to be found in *Phenomenology of Perception* (such as the "dialogue" between man and world, the concept of meaning as an "in-between" virtual phenomena, the world as an ever- moving, developing horizon and so on), the goal of this last work was to bring the insights from his early work to an

---

[1] I will not be presenting the entire philosophy of this latest work *The Visible and the Invisible* in this chapter, but only highlighting the ideas and concepts which will be of use in the psychosomatic theory developed in the later chapters of this book.

[2] This last work was only partially completed due to Merleau-Ponty's untimely death in 1961. Claude Lefort published the text posthumously in 1964, comprised of four chapters and approximately 100 pages of working notes. Merleau-Ponty seemed to have been working with these ideas from 1952 up until the time of his death. Many of the themes in this last work can be found in the collection of his lecture seminars *Themes from the Lectures at the Collège de France, 1952–1960* (1970). The article "Eye and Mind," also published posthumously in *Primacy of Perception* (1964), uses similar terminology as that found in the section "Classical Ontology and Modern Ontology" in *The Visible and the Invisible*, so it seems fair to say that these ideas were maturing in his thought during period of time. Despite the difficulties surrounding the status of posthumously published works, Merleau-Ponty's last work is an astounding text worth reading, even in its unfinished form.

J. Bullington, *The Expression of the Psychosomatic Body from a Phenomenological Perspective*, SpringerBriefs in Philosophy,
DOI: 10.1007/978-94-007-6498-9_4,

ontological level by using another starting point than the *noesis/noema* structure of phenomenology.[3] This new starting point became his notion of "the flesh[4]". In order to understand this absolutely new description of being, of which "[…] there is no name in traditional philosophy to designate it" (1964/1968, p. 139), we must keep in mind that the vision here is to render comprehensible something extremely elusive, and in order to grasp what is being described, we must follow Merleau-Ponty's thought through a labyrinth of strange terms, such as "the chiasm", "reversibility", "écart[5]/dehiscence", "the visible" and "the invisible". Where to begin? Merleau-Ponty himself begins *The Visible and the Invisible* in the following way:

> We see the things themselves, the world is what we see: formulae of this kind express a faith common to the natural man and the philosopher—the moment he opens his eyes; they refer to a deep-seated set of mute "opinions" implicated in our lives. But what is so strange about this faith is that if we seek to articulate it into theses or statements, if we ask ourselves what is this *we*, what *seeing* is, and what *thing* or *world* is, we enter into a labyrinth of difficulties and contradictions (1964/1968, p. 3).

We think we know what it is to perceive the world, nothing could be more obvious, and yet when we reflect upon it, we are forced to wonder, what does it *mean* to see? What does this seeing tell us about being, about what there is (*il y'a*)? We reach the world through our bodies (perception) but the world also reaches us. I find myself with the thing at the end of my gaze, it rests there, but it is somehow also "in me", Merleau-Ponty writes; "[…] I have in perception the thing itself, and not a representation, I will only add that that the thing is at the end of my gaze and, in general, at the end of my exploration […] I must acknowledge that the table before me sustains a singular relation with my eyes and my body: I see it only if it is within their radius of action;" (1964/1968, p. 7). How can this be understood? There is a "coupling" between the seer and the seen-thing that goes beyond the intentionality of *noesis/noema*:

> There is vision, touch, when a certain visible, a certain tangible, turns back upon the whole of the visible, the whole of the tangible, of which it is a part, or when […] between it and them, and through their commerce, is formed a Visibility, a Tangibility in itself, which belong properly neither to the body qua fact nor to the world qua fact […] since each is only the rejoinder of the other, and which therefore form a couple, a couple more real than either of them (ibid, p. 139).

---

[3] "What I want to do is restore the world as a meaning of Being absolutely different from the 'represented', that is, as the vertical Being which none of the 'representations' exhaust and which all 'reach', the wild Being" (1964/1968, p. 253).

[4] This strange term (*chair* in French) refers to the "meat" of the human body in its vulnerable, perishable nature as mortal. If this term should be understood literally or metaphorically in Merleau-Ponty's thought is debated in the literature. In any case, Merleau-Ponty's notion of the flesh should not be understood as merely referring to human bodies. He also writes about the "flesh of the world". See especially Hass (2008), Gill (1991) on the status of the term "flesh" in Merleau-Ponty's writings.

[5] The English translation of the French écart would be "divergence", "spread", "deviation", "separation".

> We understand then why we see the things themselves, in their places, where they are, according to their being which is indeed more than their being-perceived – and why at the same time we are separated from them by all the thickness of the look and of the body; it is that this distance is not the contrary of this proximity, it is deeply consonant with it, it is synonymous with it. It is that the thickness of flesh between the seer and the thing is constitutive for the thing of its visibility as for the seer of his corporality; it is not an obstacle between them, it is their means of communication (ibid, p. 135).
>
> It suffices for us for the moment to note that he who sees cannot possess the visible unless he is possessed by it, unless he *is of it* [...] (ibid, pp. 134–135).

It is this mysterious way that "we" have "the world" in a unitary movement that needs to be philosophically articulated, not in terms of phenomenology (constituting consciousness), but in terms of ontology, that is, what is the nature of being that is both us (the ones who sees) and the world (that which is seen/that which sees us)? This is the core of the flesh; that it is me and it is the world and it is always in a process of becoming. Our bodies and the world are part of the same being. We are threads in the same cloth, although the flesh of the body is not to be confused with the flesh of the world, they are not interchangeable. In fact, flesh is sustained by a "split" (dehiscence) that always keeps the human from disappearing into the things and the things from disappearing into the human, it is a unity composed of difference, held together yet kept apart.

From Lived Body to Flesh

In *Phenomenology of Perception* we saw how the notion of "dialogue" between the embodied subject and the world was described as an "intertwining". But as mentioned above, Merleau-Ponty felt that this description was still too close to the traditional phenomenological idea of meaning constitution, even if gave the body a special new role in the constitution of meaning.[6] The things were understood in *Phenomenology of Perception* as correlates of the body, but not yet in a way that satisfied Merleau-Ponty's desire to explicate the intimate bond between man and world. The system of the lived body, as mind/body unity present to the world in terms of concrete situations, worked out in *Phenomenology of Perception* gives way to a more thorough going "holism" in *The Visible and the Invisible*, where "flesh" is articulated as a temporal process wherein one and the same being turns itself back on itself and reveals both the seer and the seen in one swoop. The unfolding of the world and things is an incarnated process, and thus nature (the world) and man should be understood more like verbs than nouns. Nature unfolds itself into a human subject, who is also a bit of nature (matter), resulting in

---

6 One can however find sentences already in *Phenomenology of Perception* which precede the vision of *The Visible and the Invisible*, such as: "I understand the world because there are for me things near and far, foregrounds and horizons, and because in this way it forms a picture and acquires significance before me, and this finally because I am situated in it and it understands me" (p. 408).

nature becoming aware of itself through one of its parts. Man flows into things and things flow into man as a "chiasm",[7] a crisscrossing or reversibility that does not collapse the one into the other, but sustains both in a tension never resolved.[8] Merleau-Ponty uses an analogy from the body to illustrate this "crossing over". He refers to Husserl's famous example of the one hand touching the other.[9] We may touch our right hand with our left hand. The one hand is touching, the other hand is touched. We can then switch hands, and that which was previously touched can be the touching hand. We cannot, however, capture ourselves as the ones touching. We maintain this "split" (the toucher and the touched) in one body, and in the same way, the flesh maintains both the seer and the seen. What we call "perception" is the coiling over of the world upon itself, revealing this split that sustains the on-going scene. This division, constantly splitting and yet maintaining unity is the very being of flesh. If we were to coincide with that which we experienced, there would no longer be experience. The chiasm cannot be closed, for then all the world and all experience would collapse.

The flesh of the world and the flesh of our bodies are part of one self-dividing flesh. This reality is prior to consciousness. It is brute being, or "wild/savage being". But the flesh of the world is not the same as the flesh of the body, "The flesh of the world is not *self-sensing (se sentir)* as is my flesh – it is sensible and not sentient—I call it flesh, nonetheless [...] in order to say that it is a *pregnancy* of possibilities [...]" (ibid, p. 250). This is because the (flesh of) the world is not comprised of objects lying about, objectively in space, it is a *verb*, an event of becoming in relation to sentient beings, and in this sense, "alive". This final vision of the "in-between" is described by Merleau-Ponty succinctly in the following way:

> The flesh is not matter, in the sense of corpuscles of being which would add up or continue on one another to form beings. Nor is the visible (the things as well as my own body) some "psychic" material that would be – God knows how – brought into being by the things factually existing and acting on my factual body. In general, it is not a fact or a sum of facts "material" or "spiritual." Nor is it a representation for a mind [...] The flesh is not

---

[7] The term "chiasm" in Merleau-Ponty's text refers to the Greek "khiasmos" which means literally a crosswise arrangement. There is a grammatical meaning of chiasm as a rhetorical expression where two phrases are inversions of each other, as in: "When the going gets tough, the tough get going" or "Working hard or hardly working". Chiasm can also have an anatomical meaning referring to the crisscrossing of the optic nerve in the brain. In French, readers associate to the grammatical usage, which comes close to the concept of reversibility Merleau-Ponty was after, but in English translators have assumed that he intended the anatomical association (Evans and Lawlor 2000). Finally, the term "chiasm" has a relation to the Greek verb "chiazein" which means to mark with an X, as in the sign of the cross.

[8] "The visible about us seems to rest in itself. It is as though our vision were formed in the heart of the visible, or as though there were between it and us an intimacy as close as between the sea and the strand, And yet it is not possible that we blend into it, nor that it passes into us, for then the vision would vanish at the moment of formation, by disappearance of the seer or of the visible" (1964/1968, pp. 130–131) and "There is no coinciding of the seer with the visible. But each borrows from the other, takes from or encroaches upon the other, intersects with the other, is in chiasm with the other" (ibid, p. 261).

[9] Husserl (1989, p. 152).

> matter, is not mind, is not substance. To designate it, we should need the old term "element" in the sense it was used to speak of water, air, earth, and fire, that is, in the sense of a *general thing*, midway between the spatio-temporal individual and the idea, a sort of incarnate principle that brings a style of being wherever there is a fragment of being. The flesh is in this sense an "element" of Being (ibid, p. 139).

The flesh could thus be compared to the ancient Greeks' *arche*, that is, that *through which* things can come to be. The term flesh is by no means crystal clear, but to sum up, we find in Merleau-Ponty's notion of flesh a way to describe the coming together of man and world in the unity of upsurge (becoming together) that was not possible to describe from within a classical phenomenological framework.

The Visible and the Invisible

Let us move on to the notions of the "visible" and the "invisible". The "visible" has already been mentioned by Merleau-Ponty in the above quotations on the flesh. Hopefully, it is clear that when he speaks about the "visible" he does not mean the perceived object as such, as commonly understood, which would be too rooted in the philosophy of consciousness which he was trying to surpass in his new ontology. The visible is a completely new landscape never before articulated. It is a manner of being that comes to light as a unity of style, which is nevertheless in a constant state of transcending, it is a certain manner of "[...] managing the domain of space and time over which it has competency [...]" (ibid, p. 115). There is a kinship between the seer and the seen which opens up to each other with a familiarity that is not in the order of thought/cognition. The world is elaborated for us already. We do not "[...] look at a chaos, but at things [...]" (ibid, p. 133). What we call a visible is "[...] a quality pregnant with a texture, the surface of a depth, a cross section upon a massive being, a grain or corpuscle born by a wave of Being" (ibid, p. 136). There is familiarity to the visible, but also movement. Things come into presence but are always further on, unfolding into a horizon.[10] The domain of the flesh inaugurates this visibility for us. It is marked out because of the way in which subjects and the world partake of this unitary movement. However, the visible should not be understood as something that only has to do with our perceptual capacities:

> When we speak of the flesh of the visible we do not mean to do anthropology, to describe a world covered over with all our own projections, leaving aside what it can be under the human mask. Rather, we mean that carnal being, as a being of depths [...] is a prototype of Being, of which our body, the sensible sentient, is a very remarkable variant, but whose constitutive paradox already lies in every visible (ibid, p. 136).

---

[10] "The world is a *field,* and as such is always open" (ibid, p. 185) and "But what is proper to the visible is, we said, to be the surface of an inexhaustible depth [...]" (ibid, p. 143).

The look incorporates the seer into the visible, it is not its cause. Visibility as a result of the movement of flesh:

> There is vision, touch, when a certain visible, a certain tangible, turns back upon the whole of the visible/tangible of which it is a part, or when between it and them, and through their commerce, is formed a visibility, a tangible in itself (ibid, p. 139).

Thus, visibility is the name for that which arises when the incarnated human being and the world meet. This visibility is a visibility in general, not any particular visible thing. What is then, the invisible?

The invisible could be called the hidden perceptual ideality (a gestalt, an organized field) of the lines or forces which give structure, yet themselves remain inarticulate. The invisible regulates foreground and background, gives things their *logos*, their meaning. The invisible is the "idea" or the interior lining of things that gives both perceptual and linguistic sense. They bring meaning into play, but remain hidden themselves.

> With the first vision, the first contact, the first pleasure, there is initiation, that is, not the positing of a content, but the opening of a dimension that can never again be closed, the establishment of a level *in terms of which* [my emphasis] every other experience will henceforth be situated. The idea is this level, this dimension. It is therefore not a *de facto* invisible, like an object hidden behind another, and not an absolute invisible, which would have nothing to do with the visible. Rather, it is the invisible *of* this world, that which inhabits this world, sustains it, and renders it visible [...] (ibid, p. 151).
>
> There is a strict ideality in experiences that are experiences of the flesh: the moments of the sonata, the fragments of the luminous field, adhere to one another with a cohesion without concept, which is of the same type as the cohesion of the parts of my body, or the cohesion of my body with the world. Is my body a thing, is it an idea? It is neither, being the measurant of the things. We will therefore have to recognize an ideality that is not alien to the flesh, that gives it is axes, its depth, its dimensions (ibid, p. 152).

Thus, Merleau-Ponty locates meaning once again at a level beyond/below consciousness. The invisible renders the world visible not through constituting acts of consciousness, but by being a particular "dimension" of the visible itself. The invisible establishes levels of experiences in the same way his early notion of "structure" worked in *Phenomenology of Perception*. There is both sedimentation (the establishing of dimensions or a topography) and transformation (creation of new meanings) in the unfolding of the flesh. Certain authors have speculated that Saussure's differential or "diacritical" theory of meaning was an important inspiration for Merleau-Ponty in his later writings. According to Saussure, a signified (word) has meaning only in relation to its difference from other related signs in the whole linguistic structure. This implicit (hidden) relationship of one word to the entire edifice of language when speaking could be compared to the role of the invisible to the visible. In every visible, there is an invisible implied, in the same way that one word implies the entire language system. We do not have the entire system of language before us when we speak, but the "differences" between signs implied in language are absolutely necessary in order to speak at all. They are therefore present without being actually present (or "visible"). In a similar way, it is the invisible of the world that makes the world visible.

> Meaning is *invisible*, but the invisible is not the contradictory of the visible: the visible itself has an invisible inner framework (*membrure*), and the in-visible is the secret counterpart of the visible, it appears only within it [...] one cannot see it there and every effort to *see it there* makes it disappear, but it is *in the line* of the visible, it is its virtual focus, it is inscribed within it (1964/1968, p. 215).

One could say that the articulation of the visible and the invisible is Merleau-Ponty's solution to the problem of the dualism between perception and culture, between carnality and ideality which he grappled with during the years after *Phenomenology of Perception*. There is "meaning" or "logos" in the reversibility of flesh, where, roughly speaking, the visible could be on the "side" of materiality (the body, perception, nature) where the invisible would be on the "side" of ideality (form, structure, language, logos). One should not begin introducing dualism back into the unitary vision, but it is hard avoid some form of dualism when one is describing a unity composed of difference.

The reversibility that defines the flesh is also operating in other fields where, "[...] it is even incomparably more agile there and capable of weaving relations between bodies [...]" (1964/1968, p. 144). There exists a reversibility between different modalities of perception (sight and touch for example), between other bodies and my own, between past and present, between language and perception. For example, the intertwining of the sense modalities of the body illustrates the reversibility of difference within unity once again within the body itself (like the one hand touching the other in the previous section). To experience the coldness of a winter day engages several senses, we feel the cold air on our face when we leave the warm house, we see the frost and ice on the trees, we hear the special crunch of the snow when it is very cold. All this is united into one experience of cold weather, and yet we immerse ourselves in the one or the other sensation, switching back and forth, and this "reversibility" from sight to sound to touch shows how these modalities never coincide with each other or disappear into each other, illustrating again the chiasm of sustained difference in unity. In a similar way, we inhabit the world with others and the "intercorporeality" of the world is both my world and the world of the other. It is the same world, but I do not confuse my perspective with the perspective of the other:

> It is said that the colors, the tactile reliefs given to the other, are for me an absolute mystery, forever inaccessible. This is not completely true; for me to have not an idea, an image, nor a representation, but as it were the imminent experience of them, it suffices that I look at a landscape, that I speak of it with someone. Then, through the concordant operation of his body and my own, what I see passes into him, this individual green of the meadow under my eyes invades his vision without quitting my own, I recognize in my green his green, as the customs officer recognizes suddenly in a traveler the man whose description he had been given. There is no problem of the *alter ego* because it is not *I* who sees, not *he* who sees, because an anonymous visibility inhabits both of use, a vision in general, in virtue of that primordial property that belongs to the flesh, being here and now, of radiating everywhere and forever [...] (ibid, p. 142).

Merleau-Ponty does not want to solve "the problem of the other" through the reversibility of the flesh. He wants to transform the problem, resulting in a new idea of subjectivity. We all have primordial contact with being (the world) because we are flesh, partaking of the same movement. The other is "[...] caught up in a circuit that connects him to the world, as we ourselves are, and consequently also in a circuit that connects him to us – and this world is *common* to us" (ibid, p. 269). The "unity in difference" operating in the flesh manifests itself in the common world of human beings. We are all together in one world, although it is always *my* world that I experience, together with others. The philosophical problem of the relation of self to others would lead too far afield from our focus here. Suffice to say that Merleau-Ponty's vision of the flesh is useful on a variety of philosophical issues.

The final reversibility mentioned above is that between language and perception. Merleau-Ponty writes that the "ideal" of the flesh is made visible by its emigration into language, a "less heavy, more transparent body" (ibid, p. 153). Because we speak (see Chap. 3) the landscape is overrun by words, "as with an invasion" (ibid, p. 155), and cannot be separated from the visible. For Merleau-Ponty, "[...] there is no dialectical reversal from one of these views to the other [speech and perception]; we do not have to reassemble them into a synthesis: they are two aspect of the reversibility which is the ultimate truth" (ibid, p. 155). The structure of the human body and the movement of flesh already contain within them the possibility of language. Our existence as seers, who catch sight of one another, contains all that is needed for speech to arise, speech about the world we share, once we learn to make sounds. Just as the body and world meet in a chiasmic reversibility, so is the relationship between speech and perception. Language is not a mask over things, but the articulation of the thing, which is both perceptual (mute) and meaningful (structured).

> [...] Language is a life, is our life and the life of things. Not that *language* takes possession of life and reserves it for itself: what would there to be to say if there existed nothing but things said? It is the error of semantic philosophies to close up language as if it spoke only of itself; language lies only from silence; everything we cast to the others has germinated in this great mute land which we never leave (ibid, p. 125–126).

Language and perception are chiasmatic because we are creatures with bodies who speak. The "field" of being which we communicate with is both ideality and carnality, meaning and material. Finally the "structure" of sedimentation and spontaneous transformation which characterizes the movement of flesh is also exhibited in language. Thought and language can always transcend the sedimented meanings inscribed in the established language and culture. A new concept is formed, new turns of phrase, which in turn change the way in which we perceive the world. And this new way of seeing the world inspires further transformations of thought and language. Language is not about naming pre-existing things, putting signs on objects, but a continual articulation and transformation of the field. For example, in the tradition of painting, the expressionists suddenly "saw" light and started to paint it as they saw it, and this way of seeing suddenly became a horizon of our perception, and we could then see what they saw, or to put in another way, the expressionist style of seeing articulated a possible perspective, which became articulated, in the visible.

The last vision of Merleau-Ponty, presented in this chapter, provides a radically new way of understanding the human experience of being-in-the-world. The concepts and point of view from *The Visible and the Invisible* give us a description of the whole, thereby leaving behind our culturally ingrained way of thinking which compartmentalizes mind, body and world into separate entities. We need this picture of the whole in order to grasp the nature of psychosomatic pathology. Many patients today seek health care with complex psychosomatic symptoms which remain "medically unexplained." For this reason it is imperative that we have a complementary frame of reference with which to understand and treat these patients. The philosophical work of Merleau-Ponty can provide a fruitful point of departure for this badly needed alternative approach. His early concepts of the lived body and structure transformation as well as the later work on meaning, expression and the flesh will in the following chapters be applied to the psychosomatic problematic, resulting in a new understanding of the condition as well as providing the philosophical ground for specific treatment strategies.

References

Evans, F., & Lawlor, L. (Eds.). (2000). *Chiasms: Merleau-Ponty's notion of flesh*. Albany: State University of New York Press.

Gill, J. H. (1991). *Merleau-Ponty and metaphor*. Atlantic Highland, NJ: Humanities Press.

Hass, L. (2008). *Merleau-Ponty's philosophy*. Bloomingdale: Indiana University Press.

Husserl, E. (1989). *Ideas pertaining to a pure phenomenology and to a phenomenological philosophy, Second book: Studies in the phenomenology of constitution*. Dordrecht: Kluwer Academic.

Merleau-Ponty, M. (1945/1962). *Phenomenology of perception*. London: Routledge & Kegan Paul.

Merleau-Ponty, M. (1964). The primacy of perception. In J. M. Edie (Ed.), *The primacy of perception: And other essays on phenomenological psychology, the philosophy of art, history and politics* (pp. 12–42). Evanston, IL: Northwestern University Press.

Merleau-Ponty, M. (1964/1968). *The visible and the invisible*. Evanston, IL: Northwestern University Press.

Merleau-Ponty, M. (1970). *Themes from the lectures at the Collège de France, 1952–1960*. Evanston, IL: Northwestern University Press.

Merleau-Ponty, (1993). Phenomenology and psychoanalysis: Preface to Hesnard's *L'Oeuvre de Freud*. In K. Hoeller (Ed.), *Merleau-Ponty and psychology*. Atlantic Highland, NJ: Humanities Press.

Chapter 5
The Phenomenological Psychosomatic Theory

To be in the world as a human being means to experience the world *as* a world. As shown in the previous chapters, the notion of "experience" is reformulated in Merleau-Ponty's philosophy. Human experience (being-*towards*-the-world/*être* ***au*** *monde*) is that reversibility between man and world where both "become" in a single movement that contains a unity of difference, in a process which is ever changing and evolving over time. We are the authors of the situations we "create" just as our lived situations, in a sense, create us, and cannot be understood apart from us. There is no subject without a situation in which s/he is inserted, and no situation without a human subject for whom it is a situation. This chiasm is the creation of the meaningful world *for us*. It is the way we live the world and the way the world appears to us. Furthermore, we are creatures of habit and sedimentation, who at the same time, continually transform and surpass the given. Using the Merleau-Pontian insights of the previous chapters, the next section of this book will show how psychosomatic pathology can be understood, first and foremost, as a breakdown in the "dialogue" between man and world, reducing experience to being-in-the-world *as body*. According to the theory outlined in this book,[1] this level of meaning-constitution, the psychosomatic condition, is the result of a collapse in the natural harmony of adequate structure transformation. In psychosomatic illness, the person's sedimented structures are not adequate for handling (making sense of, containing, solving) the challenges from the life world which precipitate the psychosomatic crisis, yet the patients cannot, for various reasons, transform their structures to accommodate the challenge. Instead, the response is a rudimentary body meaning (the psychosomatic symptom), a mute signaling, which is not adequate to the task at hand. Rather than bringing thoughts, feelings, willpower, values, decision making, resoluteness and activity to the fore (meaning-constitution at the level of *self*), the person responds to the challenge at the lower end of the mind/body continuum with a body meaning. Whenever the

---

[1] I should make clear that Merleau-Ponty himself never wrote about psychosomatics. It is my own application of his concepts and insights to the phenomenon of psychosomatics which constitutes the phenomenological psychological theory presented in the following chapters.

J. Bullington, *The Expression of the Psychosomatic Body from a Phenomenological Perspective*, SpringerBriefs in Philosophy,
DOI: 10.1007/978-94-007-6498-9_5, © The Author(s) 2013

body steps in and "expresses" where higher order level meaning-constitution would be more appropriate, I call this condition "psychosomatic." This entails an altered experience of body, self and world. In the course of this chapter we will see how this is comprehensible in the light of the lived body and the flesh.

We recall that "the lived body" is the system of mind/body/world that allows for meaning (the appearance and understanding of a world) on psychosocial as well as body levels (the body also "understands" the world). There is no longer any need to worry about how the mind relates to the body. We leave the dualistic framework of traditional thinking behind and accept the description of man as an intertwining of "levels" or "planes of signification" (Merleau-Ponty 1942/1963, p. 201), which we have previously called "mind" and "body".[2] Because there is body in the mind and mind in the body, the question of "interaction" is no longer an issue. What is more interesting is the relationship between the subject, as a mind-body unity and the perceived world, between man and that upsurge of meaning that constitutes our lived experience of the world. Let us examine this relationship in terms of the sedimentation of structures and structure transformations. We can imagine that the "movement" which is the birth of human experience occurs when sedimented (bodily, mental and social) structures meet the world, a world which is already previously shaped by these very structures. These sedimented structures are in turn continuously challenged by that which they meet, as the world is always a "beyond" the already known/experienced, resulting in the transformation of structures so that structures evolve and can "take in" more and more articulated views of the world.[3] This meeting between man and world, resulting in human experience, is neither the product of a constituting consciousness (idealism) nor a passive receptivity from a ready-made world (empiricism). The meaningful human world is literally born in the encounter, as reversibility, between man and world, between a particular human subject and a concrete lived situation.

The becoming-movement of human experience, on various levels of signification, can be visualized in terms of a continuum, where the human being, constantly in a relationship to the world (in terms of concrete situations), finds him/herself on a continuum from "mind to body" such as Merleau-Ponty described in *Phenomenology of Perception.*[4] We find ourselves always in specific situations,

---

[2] I will in the following sometimes use the terms mind and body, but these should be understood as levels of the lived body , not as separate dualistic categories.

[3] This is somewhat reminiscent of Piaget's concepts of accommodation and assimilation, although here this transformation occurs on all levels, not only in terms of cognitive development.

[4] "Man taken as a concrete being is not just a psyche joined to an organism, but the movement to and fro of existence which at one time allows itself to take corporeal form and at others moves towards personal acts. Psychological motives and bodily occasions may overlap because there is not a single impulse in a living body which is entirely fortuitous in relation to psychic intentions, and not a single mental act which has not found at least its germ or its general outline in physiological tendencies" (1945/1962, p. 88).

played out at different levels of existence. Sometimes, we are in situations which engage the level of the body (*le moi naturel),* and at other times, the situation is such that it requires the level of psychosocial meaning-constitution (*the personal, psychosocial self)* in order to arise and be sustained. This movement (to and fro) on the mind/body continuum is so natural that we do not normally need to work at finding the right level in order to accommodate various situations. For example, in a teaching situation, this particular encounter between man and world will achieve its completion (be successful) if the teacher is able to bring forth and maintain the cognitive levels of the lived body. S/he will move on the mind/body continuum to that "position" where thought, speech, and communication are in the foreground. The teacher does not cease to have a body, nor even bodily experiences at that moment, but the level of the mind/body continuum which is *engaged* in this situation is primarily of the higher orders. The situation itself calls forth the level on the mind/body continuum which will make it successful. Were the teacher to abandon thought and communication and allow the body to become figure instead of ground, to use a Gestalt image, the "teaching situation" would break down, and there would be a tension or disharmony between that which was intended (the teaching situation) and the actual experienced situation, resulting in a confusing experience for both teacher and students. In this sense, the "meaning" of situations is manifested when that which is aimed for (the successful lecture) is fulfilled, through the use of adequate sedimented structures, and at times, spontaneous structure transformations, at the proper level on the mind/body continuum. For the most part, this "harmony-of-situation" works so fluidly that it is never a matter of reflection. We find ourselves at the right level at the proper time in order to make us feel at home in a variety of situations. For example, we must truly become "body" in order to fall asleep. If we think too much (too much "mind") we will not be able to fall asleep,[5] since that situation achieves its completion when the personal self recedes. In a similar way, we become "mind"/persons, for example, when being interviewed on television or radio. We will not be a successful politician if we are not able to muster up higher orders of meaning constitution when journalists ask us questions about our policies. This natural affinity between situation and mind/body response is responsible for the unproblematic flow which normally makes up meaningful human experience.

Thanks to our nature as transcending beings, we also have the capacity to initiate new situations, create new meanings and allow the world to beckon to us, arousing our curiosity and novel forms of activity. When we are in psychosomatic health, we can take in (accommodate and understand) situations which arise, as

[5] It is interesting that we say "fall" asleep in English, as the image of falling brings to mind plunging into a depth or at least losing the upright position, which is characteristic for images of personhood, such as "stand up for yourself" "to take a stand on X" "she is an upright person" etc. To lose one*self* to sleep is nothing more that relinquishing the level of mind/personhood on the mind body continuum. The same metaphor of *falling* into sleep is used in a variety of languages, such as Swedish (*falla i sömn*), Spanish (*caer dormindo*) and Ibo in Nigeria (*mmadu na- arahu ura*).

well as initiate and develop situations according to the needs and desires of our personal self. This "dialogue" between man and world is smooth and natural, even though there may arise various "tensions" in the field when one is surprised or challenged in different ways. But we can usually transform our habitual structures and find a way to continue the "dialogue" with the world.

An example of structure transformation can be illustrated by a description from the phenomenologist Kay Toombs (2001), on how her life-world became disrupted by the progressive disease of muscular sclerosis. Things she used to do without thinking, like climbing the steps up to her classroom, became impossible, and situations that were previously mastered without a thought became complicated problems to solve. A swinging door, trying to put pantyhose on immobile legs or eating a bowl of soup demanded developing new strategic ways of relating to objects. This process was by no means easy. She writes: "The surrounding world appears (feels) different than it did prior to bodily dysfunction. In particular, the world is experienced as overtly obstructive, surprisingly non-accommodating. Actions are sensed as effortful, where hitherto they had been effortless .... When ceaseless and ongoing effort is required to perform the simplest of tasks (getting out of bed, dressing, taking a shower, going on a trip), there is a powerful impulse to withdraw, to cease doing what is required. The person with a disability is tempted severely to curtail involvements in the world." (ibid, p. 253). Her habitual way of moving and perceiving no longer "worked" in these challenging situations. Learning to adapt to chronic illness and disability means learning to inhabit a new world. Transforming our ways of seeing, moving and even feeling and thinking are all a part of what it means to "cope" with challenging situations. And when we have transformed our structures, the world is a not the same. Toombs again: "I catch myself watching students running across the campus, or colleagues taking the stairs two-at-a-time, and I marvel at their effortless ability to do so. Try as I might, I can no longer remember how it was to move like that. It is not simply that I cannot recall the last occasion when I walked upright. It is that I cannot recollect, or re-imagine, the felt bodily sense of 'walking'" (ibid, p. 254).

The above illustration shows that our experiences of the world are constantly changing from the habitual/known into new articulations and nuances. Sometimes, these transformations are violent and disruptive, like finding oneself suddenly paralyzed after a car accident, or imperceptible, as when partners in a marriage gradually adapt to each other or grow apart. Because of the intimate bond between man and world as flesh, there is a reciprocal relationship that means that we are created by our situations, which we ourselves create. This folding back and forth between creating and being created is the nature of the flesh. This movement, in health, aims towards further degrees of articulation, where both the subject and the world reveal more of themselves through time. However, this same chiasm of the flesh can stagnate so that there is no movement, no articulation, no structure transformation. Situations breakdown, the self is reduced to the body and the world no longer shows any horizons to be investigated. This is psychosomatic ill health.

The Collapse in Meaning-Constitution and the Failure of Structure Transformation

Let us now examine what happens in the lived body when the psychosomatic breakdown occurs. The process begins when a challenge arises in the life of the person (suddenly or gradually over time) which would require an "answer" at the level of the self (i.e. thoughts, feelings, actions) in order to be resolved. For various reasons, this level of meaning constitution is not forthcoming, resulting in a "tension" or disharmony in the flow of experience. The challenging situation could be a marital problem, problems with child-raising, family conflicts, sexual difficulties, problems at work, economical worries or more traumatic events such as divorce, migration, death of loved ones etc. In psychosomatic health, the person would be aware of the problem and meet the challenge by reflecting, experiencing feelings and perhaps taking some kind of action in order to handle the situation. For the patient who cannot transform structures in this way, this resolution does not occur. The answer to the tension in the field of experience is to respond with a body meaning. In other words, the body starts to try to "understand" and "handle" the problem, resulting in the psychosomatic symptom.[6]

When the dialogue between man and world breaks down in this way, the only meaning-constitution that arises in relation to the challenging life situation is at the level of the body. The disruption in the flow of experience (between man and world/subject and situation) becomes transferred to and experienced in the body. Instead of focusing on the challenge, the person begins to answer the "tension" from the problematic life situation with a bodily response. In this way, the patient has reduced psychosocial problems to problems with the body. The symptom will serve as a channel for tension release, that is, it will be the "answer" to the "question" posed by the problematic life situation, but this body meaning will not resolve the tension in the lived body, which requires resolution on another level of meaning-constitution. For this reason, the unsolved problematic life situation will continue to be expressed at the level of the body, maintaining the psychosomatic symptom. At this point, the person's understanding of their predicament is lived in terms of problems with the body. This understanding becomes sedimented as the way in which they experience the world. The problem with the psychosomatic symptom is not only that the body has an "untreatable" symptom, but that the field of experience and self becomes reduced to the level of the body. The problematic body fills the experience of the world, effaces all other possible situations. The world appears only in relation to the symptom (e.g. Can I manage these stairs? How can I make it through a 3-hour meeting? and so on). There is no longer any

[6] According to this theory, no distinction is made between symptoms without material causes and symptoms with material causes. What is important is how this body symptom is *used* as a substitute for meaning-constitution on a higher level. Whether the symptom arose due to organic or psychological processes is irrelevant. Psychosomatic pathology is a way of being-in-the-world , and as such, it is how the world appears and is lived that is important.

dialogue between the patient and the world, in terms of a horizon of meaning as the give and take of reversibility described in the previous chapters. One has made oneself into a thing[7] (an obtrusive body) which blocks out all structure transformations and meaning-constitution on higher levels of articulation, leaving a depleted world and an invasive, recalcitrant body in place of a self in the "moving equilibrium" of life situations.

Clinical Examples

If we follow Merleau-Ponty in his notion of flesh, we have no problem understanding the meaning constitution involved in bodily symptoms. Indeed, even Freud understood that the body could "speak" although he lacked the philosophical framework to make this insight comprehensible. Within the context of the lived body, we may understand the psychosomatic symptom as the way in which the body "answers" the challenge from the world as a rudimentary expression. Thus, bodily levels of understanding are engaged in situations where the higher order levels are required. Instead of transforming psycho-social structures of meaning-constitution, meaning is reduced to body meaning. This results in a disarticulation of the self and world, as well as the disappearance of the transparency of the body, which is usually not the focus of our attention. To use Gestalt imagery, the body becomes figure instead of ground, ending the dialogue between man and world that constitutes psychosomatic health. I will give some clinical examples below in order to illustrate this condition.[8]

> "*Sophia*" was referred to me at the psychiatric out-patient clinic where I worked by her General Practitioner, who had come to the end of his repertoire regarding traditional somatic treatments. Sophia had an inexplicable pain that wandered in her body from her stomach to her back to her head. Her doctor told her that there was nothing more they could do for her, but that she could meet a specially trained professional at the psychiatric clinic who might be able to help her. She agreed, and arrived for her first appointment with an open, curious look on her face. She seemed to be younger than her years. On the referral from primary care, I could read that she was a divorced, middle-aged woman with two children who worked as a secretary at a medical company. I asked her to tell me about

---

[7] Sartre used the image of making oneself into a thing in his example of bad faith (*mauvais fois*) but it is not in relation to freedom that this move is made on the part of the subject according to my theory. Rather, it is the result of the breakdown of meaning constitution (structure transformation) in relation to a specific situation. The person is able to carry out habitual life activities to various degrees, but in their relation to the world as an upsurge of horizons of meaning, they have retreated from the level of self and found a "home" as an objective body. Unfortunately, health care practice often reinforced the objective body, thus sedimenting even further the experience of being a thing-to-be-repaired.

[8] All names are changed as well as non-relevant empirical data in order to protect the identity of the persons described. The cases are from my own clinical practice, my research with staff focus groups working with psychosomatic patients, or my supervision of psychosomatic casework. Illustrative cases in this chapter are taken from Bullington et al. (2003, 2005).

herself, and what she would like help with. She started out immediately by telling me about how much pain she had and how she had not been able to get any relief from medication or physical therapy. She was dissatisfied with the doctors and physical therapists she had met, convinced that they didn't take her pains seriously. And now, they have sent her to a "shrink"! She was so incapacitated by her symptoms that she was on part-time sick leave. She worked during the mornings and when she came home from work in the afternoon she had to rest in a quiet, dark room for hours in order to be in good enough "form" for when her children came home from school. This had been going on for almost a year. She hoped that I could get rid of her pains for her once and for all. I asked her why she thought that she had not been helped by medications and physiotherapy. She replied that her doctor had explained to her that her pains were related to something psychological, but she hadn't really understood what that meant. In any case, she said, the only problems she had were related to her pain. There was really no reason for her appointment with me, other than the fact that her GP had told her to come. I told Sophia that it was not that unusual that problems and worries can express themselves in the body, and that I had a great deal of experience with this kind of problem. I suggested that we meet once a week for a few months in order to see if we could try to discern what her body was "saying". I spoke about the psychosomatic connection and told her that as soon as she was able to see what her body was trying to deal with, she could resolve the problem and her body would no longer trouble her. She seemed to accept the idea, intellectually, although she had yet to be convinced that this particular kind of problem pertained to her. She didn't experience any problems other than her body symptoms. Nevertheless, she agreed to give it a try. The following week, she came to her session with a big smile on her face, sat down in the chair and began immediately recounting how much pain she had, especially after our appointment last week. It is not unusual for the first treatment session to begin in this way. Since the body has become the major mode of expression, and patients can have a feeling of demands being placed upon them in connection to the treatment plan and they will often experience symptom aggravation after the first appointment. Her tone became more complaining as she failed to evoke a response from me, and she wondered finally how on earth I could possibly be of any help? I asked her if she remembered what we had spoken of last week, about how her body has taken on the role of expression for her, she nodded, and I continued, if this is true, I wonder, what could it be that your body was trying to express after your meeting with me last week? At this point in treatment I would not expect an answer from her, but used the opportunity to reinforce the concept of the "speaking body" and show her how our work was going to take form. She shrugged her shoulders and replied that she had no idea. I assured her that what may seem difficult to understand at this point would become clearer as we moved along. I asked her to tell me what was going on in her life, besides her pain. Some patients will experience this change of focus as a rejection of their "pain story" but Sophia willingly started to tell about problems she was having at her work. She had a hard time concentrating on her tasks and found that her part-time schedule, due to her sick-leave, didn't give her enough time to do her work properly. When she came home from work, she lay down and had to rest, trying to clear the buzzing in her head, which went from worry to pain and back to worry again. She lived for her children, she said, and I understood after a time that she had few relationships, apart from her children. Her ex-husband had taken all the common friends with him when he left and she had only a few causal girlfriends whom she did not meet very often. I asked her how she felt about the friends that she lost contact with after the divorce. "How it felt? Well… it is what it is" she replied. She continued, "And I don't have time for a social life anyway, I have too much to do and too much pain". In her situation, one could imagine that she would feel anger, sorrow, feelings of loneliness and abandonment, perhaps fear and anxiety. But none of these feelings accompanied her story. That she had been abandoned by her husband and lost most of her friends had not been dealt with at the level of reflection, feelings or actions. Whenever we started to touch on such issues, she associated immediately to her pain, indeed, her body had absorbed all problems and was the cure for all ills. If only she became cured of her symptoms, everything would be all right. Instead of engaging in reflection, feelings and plans for action, she attended to her body, its symptoms, and was convinced that as soon as she got rid of the pain, everything would be "like it was before". My treatment goal was to help Sophia get back on track in terms of the "dialogue" with the world at a proper level of meaning constitution, so that her body would recede once again into the background. She needed to work through the dramatic life changes at the level of her personal self. To summarize the treatment, Sophia discovered that she had no real functioning way to contain and express anger. She came to see that in situations where she could feel anger, she felt pain instead. During the course of the treatment, she found ways that she could respond to different situations without slipping into her body expression. She became aware of rage and despair that had never been expressed in connection to her divorce. Over time, as she developed some interpersonal skills and gained confidence in herself, her body was no longer needed as a mode of expression. She became aware of how her body had "bailed her out" of difficulties, but at the price of confining her to a dark room with no real life. She was gradually able to get back to full time work, which made things actually easier for her because she could get everything done. She made some progress with activities outside of the home and her pains became less of a problem. She had learned valuable social skills which helped her become more assertive and less afraid of contact with other people. Her social life improved, and she worried less about her children and her own health.

Fadime was presented for discussion in a focus group in the context of a research project I was conducting. She was a woman in her early 30s, from a country in the Middle East, who had fled to Sweden with her husband and their child after persecution in their home country due to political activity. After several years in Sweden, her marriage fell apart and she found herself suddenly alone in a foreign country with a small child. She worked as a nurses' aid at a hospital in a large city. In connection with lifting a heavy patient, she injured her back, resulting in sick-leave from work. She was sent to various physical therapists, and received a variety of physical therapy treatments over a long period of time, without any positive results. Time passed and her doctor decided that she should have an operation. But she declined and asked to be sent to a specialized pain clinic instead, to which her doctor agreed. Since the time of the initial injury, she had developed diffuse pain in other parts of her body as well. The pain had become so intense that Fadime was bed-ridden most of the time. At the first initial appointment at the pain clinic, she appeared stiff and withdrawn. The therapist understood that Fadime had experienced many difficult things in the past, the dramatic escape from her homeland, her divorce and the demands of raising a small child in a foreign country. However, the patient didn't seem to have any emotional contact with the things she related to the therapist. She spoke of her background with an empty gaze and said with an almost inaudible voice that everything was fine except for her problems with her body. She seemed to be frozen in the chair, stiff and apparently afraid to move, so the therapist suggested perhaps joining a dance therapy movement group in order to improve body awareness and the ability to move without pain. Fadime accepted the offer, but held a very low profile during the dance therapy sessions. She performed the exercises but withdrew when the group was encouraged to investigate how they felt in connection to various movements. Fadime left the group after nine sessions, explaining that her problems were somatic in nature and she didn't see the point of the dance group, although she had liked some of the group members and looked forward to the sessions. After quitting the group, her symptoms worsened and she made appointments at the clinic with a doctor and a physical therapist. She demanded further medical treatment. Because of the multi-professional teamwork at the clinic, all the professionals who had met Fadime could agree that it was too early for the dance therapy, and she received more pain medication and acupuncture. Three months after her acupuncture treatment had finished, she contacted the original dance therapist again and asked to have individual dance therapy sessions. During the following individual therapy, she came into contact with feelings of terror, which made her tense up her body and hold her breath. She was afraid that she would literally fall apart and tried to protect her body with a rigidity and immobility which was, in fact, one of the main reasons for her muscular pain. The therapist let Fadime practice breathing into various parts of her body, using guided imagery techniques so that she could let her arms and hands relax and gradually move her arms and legs (sitting in a chair) without experiencing pain and terror. Grounding techniques helped the patient become aware of stability and contact with the ground and the seat which held her body safely. Working from the perimeter towards the center of the body, the therapist tried to help Fadime experience her back as stable yet relaxed. Unfortunately, when the focus approached the back, the patient once again left the therapy, stating one more time that her problem were somatic and she had no reason to come to the therapist. She said that she needed to find some medically sound way to get rid of her pain. Even before higher order levels of meaning constitution were intimated, the patient could not stand the provocation of lessening her muscle defences in her back. However after a few months, Fadime once again took contact with the therapist and asked to join the dance group again. She told the therapist that she now realized that her symptoms had something to do with her life situation, and she wanted to try to understand what her body was trying to tell her. As her fear of pain was worked through and her rigidity relaxed, she came into contact of with feelings of sorrow over her father's death, mourning over the loss of her home country, and existential reflections about life and death. When she could formulate these issues, she became more coordinated and stronger in her body, her voice became louder. She knew that she would not break apart if she moved and breathed and spoke up. After 20 sessions of group therapy and 12 complementary individual therapy sessions, the treatment was finished. Fadime had decided to take up her academic studies which she had been forced to leave in connection with her flight to Sweden. She never called the clinic again for an appointment after the completion of her therapy.

Kathy was being treated at an out-patient psychiatric ward where I held regular supervision on psychosomatic cases. This 40-year old woman had been a victim of incest for many years while growing up, her first rape by her father occurring when she was only 8 years old. The occupational therapist working with her (here called Mary) had Kathy in one of her rehabilitation groups and in an individual therapy treatment. The goal was to try to get her back to work after a long period of sick leave. Individual therapy with the occupation therapist and participation in the same therapists' rehab group was the basic treatment strategy that had been going on for about 2 months when Mary took up Kathy's case in supervision. Kathy had been on sick-leave for over 2 years from her work as a salesperson because of stomach problems. She had been a well functioning competent person until she had suddenly fallen apart and become a "basket case" as she herself put it. She had no clue as to what happened to her, but Mary had put together that the breakdown had occurred a short time after a re-organization at the workplace. Kathy suddenly found herself working with completely new co-workers and Mary suspected that this situation had triggered her illness. Kathy had been thoroughly examined somatically and there were no organic reasons for the violent stomach pains and elimination problems that tortured her. She was not particularly interested in her treatment at the psychiatric clinic, but came to her appointments since it was the condition for her continued sick-leave from work. She had started to develop phobias recently and told Mary that she didn't want to come to the rehabilitation group any more. Mary related how Kathy often left the group during cooking or painting or whatever activity was going on. She went into another room and stayed there by herself. She had told Mary about her traumatic past, but without showing any signs of wanting to do any therapeutic work. She spoke mainly about her stomach. Mary had tired of hearing about the stomach problems and wondered how this rehabilitation could move forward? What if she leaves the group? What can we talk about besides her stomach? I asked Mary what she herself felt in her own body when she thought about Kathy's stomach pains. Mary reflected a moment and replied "overwhelmed." She associated further that she got an image of a boundless, powerful, cascading wall of water that never stopped, enveloping her on all sides. She tensed her own body to try to get rid of the feeling of powerlessness against this relentless force. We imaged that this could be Mary's own body tuning into Kathy's experiences of vulnerability and inability to protect her body from the abusive, sexual invasion from her father. We started to discuss Kathy's inability to keep boundaries, and Mary confirmed that whenever Kathy felt irritated or provoked, she left the room, as if the only way to contain her feelings were to physically remove herself from the source. We then wondered how Kathy had felt when all her colleagues were new for her. If she had problems with setting boundaries, it may be that the job situation was too "overwhelming" for her, and she had not been able to cope with so many unknown persons at one time. Her inability to protect herself from her co-workers had activated memories and feelings from the years of abuse that she had not succeeded in containing. The body was trying to help her with these feelings and memories, but was not able to resolve this tension. These issues from the past were so powerful that even when she was taken away from the work place, the body continued in its expression in the attempt to "close the Gestalt" and be liberated from the past. So, how to go on from here? I suggested that if Kathy could not approach her trauma through verbal therapy, it may be a good idea to try another therapy form, such as art therapy, which the occupational therapist was competent to work with. The occupational therapist was positive to the suggestion of art therapy, and said that she was going to be more aware of boundary issues in the group setting and see if she could work with Kathy in order to help her feel safe about her boundaries in relation to other people in the group. At the next supervision, Mary related how she had asked Kathy to draw a picture of herself, in any situation she wanted. Kathy had drawn herself surrounded by various figures very close to her in the middle of the page. She had no feet in the picture and seemed to float in the air. Kathy said that she felt very frightened and alone in this picture. After this first picture, a whole series around this theme emerged, and Kathy was able to talk about the pictures in a much freer way than she had spoken about herself directly. Eventually, the time around the psychosomatic breakdown became clear for Kathy. She explained to Mary that she had felt "strange" and uncomfortable the months before her collapse. When she had before simply dismissed this period as "a bad time" she could now articulate specific incidents and how she felt about them. The theme of being overwhelmed was a description that Kathy could relate to, and from this phase onward Mary felt that Kathy was "onboard." Mary was not as accepting when Kathy left group, and encouraged her to stay and work with what she was thinking and feeling when she got an impulse to leave the room. After 6 months, Kathy was able to go back to work part-time. She had a found a way to understanding her stomach pains and no longer fixated on them as something that someone else needed to fix, but rather as valuable clues about what she needed to work on in order to cope with her past and present life situation.

Hawa was a middle-aged woman originally from a country in the Middle-East who was referred to our psychiatric out-patient clinic because of somatic symptoms which could not be explained by any organic causes. She felt that her arms became very tired, heavy and warm. She got so exhausted by this she had to lie down. She could be in bed for several days at a time, until her symptoms abated. She said that she felt paralyzed in her arms and was incapable of doing anything during the time she felt her symptoms. She did not work outside the home, but had a large family to take care. When she felt these symptoms, she was incapable of doing housework and her oldest daughter had to shop and cook and clean. This bothered Hawa, since she understood that it was a burden for her teen-aged daughter, who would rather be doing other things with her friends. Hawa was married, but could not imagine that her husband could help with the chores. She told me that men simply did not do such things where she came from. She laughed out loud at the thought of him hanging up laundry. She spoke with great emphasis about how terrible her situation was, with her paralyzed arms. I quickly got the picture of the paralyzed arms as a protest against her wife and mother duties of day to day life. I understood that she was tired doing all of the housework, but she lacked higher order structures with which to express this dissatisfaction. Her paralyzed arms got her out of the chores, but the price was to inflict work on her daughter, which gave rise to guilty feelings. The problem could have been easily solved by asking her husband to help out at home, but that was not an option for her. The arms she needed in order to cook and clean were out of order, but this "solution" gave her no peace. How to begin to introduce the psychosomatic connection with Hawa? She had already met a variety of specialists over the years. It was not her wish to be sitting with a therapist at a psychiatric clinic, but this was all her GP could suggest. She had felt badly treated and misunderstood in her previous clinical encounters. No one was competent enough to find out what was wrong with her, no one took her seriously. She asked me how it was possible that we had such terrible health care education here in Sweden, doctors didn't seem to know anything at all. After she had finished telling me how horrible her situation was, she looked at me with a sceptical expression and asked what I had to offer. I thought that it would be best to go right to the body, and I told her we were going to do some exercises today. After listening to her, I saw no opening for trying to discuss the psychosomatic connection. I said that I wanted to see if she could relax and wanted to ask her about how she experienced her body here and now. She replied that she was not tense. I said that she had not been helped by any medication or traditional physiotherapy, so we needed to explore how she experienced her body. She went along and closed her eyes. During the exercise (progressive relaxation in sitting position) I saw that she had very little contact with her muscles and when I asked her how she felt, she replied "nothing special". After we finished I asked her if she noticed if her symptoms were more bothersome in certain situations rather than others? She said that she felt worse during certain weather conditions, after eating certain foods and after performing certain physical chores. I thanked her and welcomed her back the following week. She came to the second session with a heavy step and sunk into the chair and looked at me with tired eyes. Her whole demeanor was passive and waiting. I asked her if we could examine the chores which made her become paralyzed in her arms. I tried to interest her in a connection between something *she* did and her symptoms so that she could see herself not just a passive victim, but as someone who could actually do something about her condition. She answered my questions shortly, always ending by looking at me inquisitively, with tired eyes. After half the session, she came back to the question of why no one could give her a diagnosis. She associated to her daughter and started to cry. How could we let her daughter suffer like this, if not for her sake, then at least for her daughter we should make an effort to cure her. It was outrageous. That she herself was the cause of this burden for her daughter and the feelings that aroused in her were displaced into a vigorous attack on me and the rest of the health care system. When she was finished, I decided to try again with the alternative of the husband helping out. This was, of course, a ridiculous idea. If he did such things, she would not consider him to be a man. She wanted to take care of her husband, children and home, she assured me. It was just that there was something wrong with her arms. We meet for a few more sessions, but the working alliance was never established. I could not interest her in the "speaking" body, and she couldn't make me fix her "objective" body. I had not been able to find a way to communicate the psychosomatic treatment, so we parted, agreeing that there was nothing I could offer her.

Let us now examine the above clinical cases in light of the phenomenological psychosomatic theory. If we recall the concept of the intentional arc from *Phenomenology of Perception* we find a description of that function which gives us our whole existence at one sweep; the past, the future, myself, my bodily "I can", my understanding of every situation, instantaneously. It is the "setting of our lives" that is a given for us. This "being-situated" is accomplished thanks to the movement in the chiasm of human experience which allows the world to "address" me in both habitual and novel ways. Likewise, there is, in me, a facility and competence that allows me to answer this world and even ask the world my own "questions" from the point of view of the personal self (interests, desires and so on). This is our ordinary way of being and we lack awareness of this chiasm because we take it for granted as "the world." In the patient examples above, something has disturbed this natural harmony and resulted in the development of psychosomatic symptoms. For example, Sophia suffered a dramatic life change when her husband left the marriage and she lost most of her social network. The challenge for her would have been to transform her structures (her feelings and understanding of her situation) so that they would be able to "harmonize" with that new life situation. The old structures could no longer accommodate what she was facing. To cope with this situation she needed to change her view of herself, her husband, her marriage, parenting, and social life. She would have needed to feel a variety of strong emotions, recognize them and contain them by allowing them to be expressed and gradually transformed into her life experience. Her entire "intentional arc" had to be readjusted so that she could continue to act and think and feel in this new situation. But because she could not do this, her body attempted to resolve the problem. This "work" of the body gradually effaces the things the world "affords". The downward spiral of somatisation is the gradual dis-articulation of the field of experience. All situations are reduced to body and habit. Sophia did not reflect on her situation or feel anything in connection to it, she simply found herself for the most part in the habitual, i.e. taking care of her work, her children and spending the rest of her time lying down in a dark room with no stimuli to disturb her.

Fadime had likewise not been able to accommodate her life situation with her habitual structures, and had not been able to transform her structures in order to cope. The world presented itself to Fadime in terms of a nameless terror that she suppressed by muscular tension and a fixation with her back injury. The "expression" of her predicament was not "I am afraid, I feel alone, I mourn my father, I miss my home country, I worry about being able to support myself and my child" but rather, a back pain, which started out as an injury but developed into a rudimentary expression of all that which she could not express through higher order structures. In order to achieve a meaning-constitution at an adequate level, Fadime needed help in order to break the somatic muscular defence, feel the strong emotions that were demanding expression, and give all of this a "meaning" that allowed her to further articulate herself and her experience the world. The failure of structure transformation and the concomitant breakdown in meaning-constitution at the proper level initiates a levelling down of experience that is characteristic of the "field" for these patients. The clinical challenge for from the point of view of this theory of psychosomatics is how to help the patient get from body expression back to personal, higher order meaning-constitution.

The phenomenological theory of psychosomatics is not designed to identify general "factors" which are responsible for psychosomatic pathology, and it is not possible to formulate any universal reasons for this inability to transform structures. Some psychosomatic patients have been previously well-functioning before their break down, others have been struggling with psychosomatic tendencies all their lives. Often, they have not been able to develop their structures due to overwhelming incidents they experienced as children, which were never formulated in terms of higher order meaning-constitution, as they were not mature enough at the time to accomplish such structure transformations. Some patients have grown up a family where the expression of one's own inner life (thoughts, feelings, opinions differing from the parents) was discouraged or even punished. For whatever reason, that which shows itself as an adult is the inability to engage higher order meaning-constitution at the level of the psycho-social self in various challenging life situations. In this sense, the psychosomatic solution could be said to be a retreat from the personal self. To be a self is to be in a process of becoming, where one's sense of self and experience of the world are continually transformed, in interaction with other people and various life situations. When this task becomes too difficult, the body steps in and lower order body meaning replaces meaning-constitution at the level of the self. When we meet these patients, we find a person who has left the arena where the self can become, presenting intractable somatic symptoms, a fixation on the body solution, a lack of awareness of any challenge from their lives and an unwillingness or inability to view the symptoms as anything other than a medical problem that needs to be fixed by health care professionals. The path to psychosomatic health resides not in fixing the body, but rather in helping the patient reinstate the "reversibility" between the subject and his/her life situation. They are stuck at the level of the body and because this solution leads to a levelling down of both self and world, they need help to get back on track.

It may seem at a first glance that the clinical examples given above could very well come from the tradition of psychosomatic medicine, with the basic assumption that strong emotions are the cause of psychosomatic pathology. It is indeed often the case that emotions (or rather, the inability to experience, contain and express emotions) play a part in the psychosomatic breakdown. However, the phenomenological theory outlines here is based on Merleau-Pontian insights, and when we say that the patient needs to "express" feelings, we mean expression in terms of the human beings innate capacity to transcend the given and move forward to new horizons in the reversibility that is the flesh. "Expression" has an existential meaning in this theory of psychosomatics, as expression is the fulfilment of our nature as human beings in our ability to maintain the dialogue with the world in the reciprocal process of becoming that is the flesh. Thus, sense-making and the development of the personal self are not luxuries for the privileged, but part of our very being. Thus, psychosomatic ill health must be understood existentially.[9] When we no longer partake of that moving equilibrium which is the

[9] Medard Boss has used insights from Heidegger to form his own existential form of psychoanalysis called *Dasein analytic*. This therapy is based on the Heideggerian notions of *Dasein* (being-there), being-towards-death, anticipatory resoluteness and so on. Although Boss criticizes both Freudian theory and psychosomatic medicine for reasons similar to my own, his

human experience of meaning, and become fixated as a thing-body, we are truly not at home, not our*selves*. So the problem with psychosomatic symptoms is ultimately a problem of being-in-the-world, an alienation from one's self and the world as movement and reversibility between man and world (situation) in the reciprocal creation of meaning. For this reason, the treatment of this condition needs another framework than the biomedical treatment of the objective body.

The Treatment[10]

That which brings the patient to a health care professional is a somatic symptom which expresses the patient's disrupted lived body. The body has become an obtrusive thing which blocks out all "dialogue" with the world. The precipitation of this condition is a challenge that has not been possible to handle with sedimented structures and the person has not been able to transform structures to meet the challenge at the appropriate level. The patient will be more or less hostile to the suggestion that the answer to their problem lies elsewhere than traditional medical treatment. However, their somatic symptoms do not abate after the usual medical repertoire. Because the patients are not initially amenable to any form of psychotherapy, they find themselves truly in a no man's land. This means that the first phase of the treatment must be about re-defining the problem from a body problem to a life-world problem. The patients do not need to understand Merleau-Ponty's notion of the lived body, but they must be willing to let go of the hope that the cure will ultimately be found at the somatic level. This initial redefinition phase serves three functions; (1) to give the patient an intellectual understanding of the mind–body connection, (2) to remove the stigmatization connected to psychosomatic conditions, and (3) to give the patient the hope of recovery. This phase is pedagogical in nature and absolutely necessary in order for the patient to be willing to come to the sessions. As long as they still harbour hopes of a strictly somatic cure, they will not persevere in the treatment.

When the patient has agreed to the treatment strategy, the next step is to help the patient experience the connection between the psychosomatic symptom and

(Footnote 9 continued)
alternative is different from mine. We are both concerned with being-in-the-world and the body, but the concepts and categories of understanding used by Boss diverge from the understanding presented here. See Bingswanger (1975), Boss (1979) and van Deurzen and Kenward (2005) for literature from this tradition.

[10] The approach described in this section bears a certain resemblance to the so-called "reattribution theory" (Dowrick et al 2008), which aims at helping the patient understand the links between physical symptoms and psychosocial issues. Although there are studies that indicate that clinicians find training in reattribution to be useful, there is no consensus on the value of reattribution for patients. There could be several reasons for this. My position is that reattribution theory has not taken into consideration the complexity of meaning constitution, having focused primarily on the cognitive level.

their life situation, so that "psychosomatic" becomes not only an intellectual concept but a lived reality. This is difficult, because the patient has been focused on the body for such a long time that there is little else present in their field of experience, except the habitual, lived out in a dis-articulated field. Nevertheless, it is possible to find these connections. One way is to ask the patient to keep a diary every day, and instruct them to write down when they experienced their symptoms as most bothersome, and when they experienced them as least obtrusive during the day. They are also instructed to write down what they were doing at these times, so that a life-world story begins to appear. The descriptions will not be very detailed in the beginning, but the therapist and the patient go through the dairy every week, and the therapist asks questions in order to help the patient articulate more and more of what they experience during their days. The descriptions of symptoms gradually give way to descriptions of the patient's life. After a time, patterns emerge, where the patient can see that s/he experiences her symptoms at their worst when there is something specific going on, like an obligatory phone call to the mother, or going to work, or meeting a certain person or anticipating being in a certain situation and so on. Week after week, the evidence builds up and the patient finally discovers a key to understanding what her body is expressing. As therapist, one listens to the blanks in the life-world story that are filled by the symptom, asking oneself "What would be there if the symptoms were not?" "What is it that the patient is having difficulty articulating on higher levels of meaning?" Another way of approaching the meaning-constitution of the body is to work directly with the body. As illustrated in the case of Fadime, it may be necessary to do body work before the patient is ready to accept the psychosomatic treatment. Body-awareness training and relaxation techniques can help the patient accept the body and in many cases remove the fear that is connected to the body and the symptom. If the patient has difficulty reflecting and putting things into words, alternative non-verbal therapy forms can be a good way to build up a working alliance so that the patient can open up to new meanings, even if they remain at the level of the body (i.e. to move in a new way, sit in a new way, feel one's body in a new way) or if emotions are experienced first in the music or in the picture, as in the example from music therapy below:

> A Swedish man in his 30s came to the clinic because of pain in his neck, shoulders, back and upper extremities. He had neurological symptoms without certain organic cause, and part of his treatment at the clinic was music therapy. Although his initial attitude was that he did not "believe in" music therapy, he consented to give it a try. He had a complicated childhood, growing up with an alcoholic parent. At the beginning of therapy, it was obvious that his main emotion was hate. He was not able to express many other feelings. The images and associations he had to various types of music were often about heroic action and battlefields showing his preoccupation with violence and conflict. Although he was extremely occupied with these types of images, in his own life he was incapable of dealing with conflicts in a constructive way. His typical behavior was usually to flee in panic in the face of potential conflicts. During one therapy session, while listening to music, he noted with surprise that he felt a feeling of peace and harmony coming from the music. He could not experience this feeling within himself, but had a clear sense of this feeling in the music. Although he could eventually admit that he was indeed experiencing strange new feelings in the therapy room, he maintained that he could never experience such feelings outside

therapy, in the "real world." However, after 20 weekly sessions of music therapy, he was not only able to experience a variety of feelings in the therapy sessions. He could also feel his feelings in his own life outside of therapy. He used the music in order to experience different feelings. He learned that he could face up to conflicts without running away, admit when he was wrong and apologize for himself when called for. He returned to significant geographical places, first not daring to get out of the car. But after awhile he could leave the car, walked about, breathe the air and remember episodes from the past. He began to forgive himself and others. When these new aspects of life opened up for him, he often laughed or expressed a profound feeling of surprise. He came to understand that feelings were in him, not only in the music, that he could have all sorts of feelings in his "real life." He was gradually able to handle conflicts and take responsibility for himself. All of these insights helped him to heal his self—image as well as his painful body. His symptoms decreased and hatred no longer dominated his emotional life.

When the patient has discovered that the body is trying to "speak" they become interested in the messages conveyed. A process of articulation is started on all levels. They can experience their bodies as both disturbing but also as transparent, that is, receding into the background, at least for short periods of time. The process of articulation helps them differentiate between different feelings, between the past and the present (often traumatic experiences remain the "invisible" lining of the present), between themselves and other persons. The world becomes filled with possibilities to be explored and the self is freed to continue to develop in the on-going dialogue with the world.

The most important therapeutic attitude on the part of the therapist is to be able to listen to the patients' level of meaning-constitution without, on the one hand, further sedimenting the psychosomatic expression (i.e. staying at the level of the body) nor moving too quickly (too much "mind") so that the patient terminates the treatment. The balance is to find a way to transform body meaning into personal meaning in small steps. The therapist has two pre-suppositions when meeting the patient, (1) meaning-constitution is stuck at the level of the body, thus hindering the resolution of a "tension" in the lived body between the patient and his/her world, (2) the patient experiences a dis-articulated field (nothing is really "there") and as such, the dialogue between the patient and her situations has broken down. Her experience of her body has blocked out the reversibility of the flesh, and she has reduced herself to a body-thing. With these two insights we may conclude that the treatment must transform body meaning to personal meaning through structure transformation and the patient must allow the body to recede into the background so that situations can arise and meaning-constitution at the level of the personal self can be reinstated. So, the psychosomatic way of being-in-the-world must be jarred out of sedimentation in order for the patient to be cured. This process can differ from case to case, but generally the road to recovery can be said to be made up of structure transformation at the level of perception, affect and sense of self. The first transformation that must occur is on a perceptual level, that is, what is the patient experiencing perceptually? What does the world "afford" them in terms of cues and invitations to be explored? Because they are living with habitual, rigid structures, nothing new is "seen". They may pass a wonderful park in the autumn, with a beautiful play of sunlight on the leaves of the trees and not "see" it. An adorable child may sit in front of them on the subway, a sumptuous meal placed before them. None of these things are experienced *as* beautiful, as adorable, as sumptuous. The world hides its splendor and does not show itself to the person who is living in the dis-articulated field of body-meaning. In order to *find* one has to *look*. So at the level of perceptual experience, the patients need to learn how to look again. This exercise of taking a conscious focus on the quality of things and experiences is a way to break the dominance of the habitual and move the focus of experience from body to world. The more one looks, the more one finds, and the more one finds, the more one is inspired to keep looking. So, opening up the senses to the world as a world with qualities and different perceptual experiences is a step towards the re-articulation of the field. When the patient starts to look for and find things, the dominance of the habitual and the body has been broken. This may be accomplished through the diary work described above, or homework which the patient does between sessions. The patient will not naturally focus on the world pole of the lived body, so they must make a special effort.

The second transformation that must be made is at the level of affect.[11] The patients often have difficulties formulating and feeling emotions, accepting and containing them. For this reason, structures must be developed in order to handle the emotional aspects of life-situations, especially the challenging life-situation that is "feeding" the psychosomatic symptom. This is also a matter of articulation for the patient, i.e. *what* is felt, *when* and *how* and for *what reasons*. Often, the symptom is replacing an emotion, so the movement from body meaning to personal higher order meaning has to do with the articulation of affect in specific situations. When situations become salient and feelings are expressed, the experience of self and world is gradually transformed. When the patient can look for, find and experience a variety of situations, and is able to feel and contain emotion in connection to them, meaning-constitution has been reinstated at the higher order level of the personal self. The patients have a better grasp of who they are, what they want and how to go about obtaining it. When this stability is achieved, it will be easier for them to work with the problematic life situation that cast them into the body-solution. Not uncommonly, a resoluteness and feeling of taking responsibility for oneself follows the re-instatement of higher order meaning-constitution. At this point, the reversibility of the flesh has opened up the dialogue between man and world and psychosomatic health is reinstated. This does not mean that the therapy is finished, there may be issues that need to be worked through, as in any psychotherapy, but the psychosomatic way of being-in-the-world has been transformed and the patient is free to work with their problems as any other patient in psychotherapy.

[11] There are a variety of techniques available to work with affect, both body-oriented (affect focused body psychotherapy) and psychotherapeutic. See Downing (1994), Monsen and Monsen (1999, 2000) and Tomkins' affect imagery consciousness (AIC) (1962, 1963).

Teaching and Supervising

Different health care professionals come into contact with patients who have psychosomatic health problems in a variety of health care settings. Some professionals have the training and the proper setting in order to be able to treat these patients at their place of work, others meet them in a context where it is not possible to offer a psychosomatic treatment plan on site. Regardless of where the professional is working, all health care staff needs to have an understanding of psychosomatics, since a great number of patients seek health care for these kinds of health problems (see Chap. 1). The initial phase of redefinition (from body problem to life-world problem) can be performed by all professionals who have contact with the patient, regardless of setting. However, because of the delicate nature of this phase, this takes certain skills and sensibilities. How can one teach students at the undergraduate level about psychosomatics and prepare them for being able to motivate the patient to an adequate treatment?

In order to convey an intellectual understanding of the mind–body connection, the student has to have an understanding of the lived body. They do not have to read Merleau-Ponty's texts, but they do need to understand that the "objective" body that they study in their anatomy books is not the primordial, lived body of the patient who is suffering. Patients do not experience low levels of serotonin, they experience being depressed, which has its own way of being lived through. The students need to understand that the way we experience our bodies influences the way we experience ourselves and the world around us. An exercise in order to raise awareness about this can be to ask the students to keep a diary of their experiences next time they are ill. When they get a cold, the flue, a headache or muscle pains, ask them to be very attentive to how they are influenced by this condition and write everything down. How are do their thoughts and actions differ compared to when they are healthy? How do they experience themselves, and others? Even a slight bout of ill health, if examined properly, can give insights into the holistic nature of the lived body. The body, self and world are intertwined, and this must be the starting point for an understanding of psychosomatics. Reading classical literature is another way to get students in the health-care professions to develop their understanding of the lived body.[12] The risk is that if the education course work is mainly focused on the objective body, it is easy to forget that this objective body is never the body they encounter in the clinic. The patient will be Mr. Grey and Ms. Jones and Mrs. Knight. Another important aspect of training for students would be to ask them to examine their own attitudes towards psychosomatic patients. What do they think about them? Some students may have worked previously at a work place that had a jargon of contempt or humor about these patients. It is important to lift such prejudices into the light for examination. The next question is, how can they convey both acceptance of the patient in their

[12] See Ahlzéns doctoral dissertation, *Why should physicians read: Understanding clinical judgment and its relation to literary experience* (2010).

psychosomatic condition as well as being able to motivate them to a psychosomatic treatment strategy? If appropriate, the students can receive supervision during their clinical placements and learn to identify their own reactions to these patients, as well as practice pedagogical skills in conveying knowledge about the mind–body connection. Many health care educations have a course or an elective on communication skills, empathetic listening and the like. It would be easy to include the clinical encounter with psychosomatic problems in such a course. A video-taped roll play between two students, one playing the role of the professional and other the role of the patient with psychosomatic health care problems, can serve as an initial way of introducing this theme, using the tapes as a starting point for seminar supervision and discussion.

Supervision for staff often has to do with the professionals' inability to connect with the patient with psychosomatic symptoms and move forward in the therapy process. The problem is usually either that the communication remains at the level of the body, where the therapist/health care professional tires of hearing about the somatic symptom time and again, or the patient threatens to leave the therapy when it moves too quickly (for example, Fadime's case). The professionals need help initiating the structure transformation process without scaring off the patient. The scenario could be a physical therapist who cannot motivate his patient to a psychosomatic treatment, or a psychologist who feels that the patient's body symptoms are standing in the way of working through feelings and painful memories, or a medical doctor who says that she has nothing to offer a patient who will not give up in their quest for a medical solution to their problem. That which all these scenarios have in common is that whatever the professionals have in their usual treatment repertoire, it is not working. Something else is required. Those professionals seeking supervision or education about psychosomatics are often experienced clinicians who have discovered that they need a new approach in order to successfully treat these patients. The most common questions I have received during my supervision are: How can you just sit and listen week after week to someone who only wants to talk about their symptoms? What should you do when you have nothing to offer the patient? Is there trauma so difficult that it is impossible to verbalize? Should one even try? How can you motivate someone to examine their life when all they want to do is examine their body? The stagnation of the treatment can be a great challenge to the self-esteem of the professional. They may be constantly criticized and attacked by the patient, and there is a great temptation to give up. When this stagnation becomes apparent to the therapist, it is good idea to get supervision to see if the case can be managed. The basic problem is for the most part that they have not been able to perform the necessary redefinition work. However, if the patient does not feel confidence and trust in the therapist/professional, this work will be difficult to accomplish. In such cases, it is often advisable to work with the body if the patient has great difficulty accepting the psychosomatic connection. The patient needs to be encountered at the level where they are expressing, which is, for the time being, the body symptom. To work with the body, when the patient presents the body as the problem, helps the patient to feel accepted and taken seriously. The therapist does not need to embrace the idea of a somatic solution in order to work with the body. One can work through the body to open up new horizons of experience. For example, one can help the patient experience their body in different ways, which can break up rigid, habitual ways of moving and feeling. If the patient feels that s/he can have some degree of control over the body it will lessen the fear and reduce their anxiety. It may happen that one may have a breakthrough to the level of personal meaning during a session of body work (a thought, feeling or memory) in connection to an exercise, and the patient may be willing to share it with the therapist. For the therapist, it is important to rest in the assurance that structure transformation is possible. This will give the proper, calm perspective needed when the patient is attacking or questioning one's competence. One must try to be open and flexible in the encounter, avoiding all impulses towards being clever and insightful. A common experience in a focus group I lead was the interesting fact that the staff reported that patients often said something of vital importance in the very last minutes of the therapy. What could this mean? Did it mean that the patient didn't want to wait around to see the therapist's reaction? The group came to another conclusion, namely, they found that these important moments occurred when they had already "ended" the session for their part. They had stopped being clever, stopped trying to "understand", stopped "doing things", at which point a freedom had opened up in the room which the patient immediately used in order to make progress. If one can establish this kind of freedom in oneself during the entire session, it can be easier to establish contact with the patient. Since they have often been rejected and dismissed from health care so many times before, just the fact of sitting with them during the sessions and not trying to get rid of them can convey a message of hope to the patient, even if they don't verbalize it as such.

When one has established contact, the patient feels comfortable and trusting. At this point, they may have accepted, at least in theory, the psychosomatic explanation for their troubles. When this redefinition of their problem is completed, one can get on with the work of listening to what the body is trying to say. As mentioned previously, there are a variety of techniques and alternative therapy forms which can be used. The progress in the therapeutic process will be marked by the patient's ability to *see/experience* more, *feel* more and eventually *do* more as the spell of the body is lifted. When staff bring patient work to supervision it is often because they are having problems establishing contact. Sometimes, one simply can't get through to the patient (like the example of Hawa) and here it is just a matter of accepting that this sometimes happens and it is all right and even proper to end the treatment. At other times, the therapist has simply become frazzled and nervous about the case, feeling tempted to quit. In this case, it will be enough to just relax, trust in one's own competence and work on building an alliance with the patient, at whatever level this is possible. This will of course take different forms for the different health care professionals, but in the cases I have supervised, when one gets a better understanding of the difficulties the patient is dealing with, it is easier to contain the "symptom talk" in the confidence that given the right therapeutic alliance this body meaning will eventually transform into personal meaning, giving the patient back both a world and a self.

This chapter has illustrated how insights from Merleau-Ponty's work can give a new perspective on psychosomatic pathology. I will in the next chapter examine the bigger picture of health and illness from a truly "holistic" perspective grounded in the phenomenology of the flesh. The scientific literature of the day is full of references to "holistic care" and "holistic medicine" but one rarely sees any real content to this term, except for some empty phrases about man being a biological, psychological social being. I believe that a sound holistic view of health can be extrapolated from the theory of psychosomatics, which should be an appreciated contribution to the literature on health.

References

Ahlzén, R. (2010). *Why should physicians read? Understanding clinical judgment and its relation to literary experience*. Dissertation of University of Durham, Universitetstryckeriet, Karlstad.

Binswanger, L. (1975). *Being-in-the-world. Selected papers of Ludwig Binswanger*. London: Souvenir Press.

Boss, M. (1979). *Existential foundations of medicine and psychology*. New York: Aronson.

Bullington, J., Nordemar, K., Nordemar, K., & Sjöström-Flanagan, C. (2003). Meaning out of Chaos: A way to understand chronic pain. *Scandinavian Journal of Caring Sciences, 17*, 325–331.

Bullington, J., Sjöström-Flanagan, C., Nordemar, K., & Nordemar, K. (2005). From pain through chaos towards new meaning: two case studies. *The Arts in Psychotherapy, 32*(14), 261–274.

Downing, G. (1994). *The body and the word*. New York: Routledge.

Dowrick, C., Gask, L., Hughes, J. G., Huw, C. J., Hogg, J. A., Peters, S., Salmon, P., Rogers, A. R., Morriss, R. K. (2008). General practitioners views on reattribution for patients with medically unexplained symptoms: a questionnaire and qualitative study. *BMC Family Practice*, *9*:46, open access.

Merleau-Ponty, M. (1942/1963). *The structure of behavior*. Boston: Beacon Press.

Merleau-Ponty, M. (1945/1962). *Phenomenology of perception*. London: Routledge & Kegan Paul.

Monsen, J. T., & Monsen, K. (1999). Affects and affect consciousness: a psychotherapy model integrating Silvan Tomkin's affect and script theory within the framework of self psychology. In A. Goldberg (Ed.), *Pluralism in self psychology: Progress in self psychology* (Vol. 15, pp. 287–306). Hillsdale: Analytic Press.

Monsen, K., & Monsen, T. J. (2000). Chronic pain and psychodynamic body therapy. *Psychotherapy, 37*, 257–269.

Tomkins, S. (1962). *Affect, imagery, consciousness, the positive affects* (Vol. 1). New York: Springer.

Tomkins, S. (1963). *Affect, imagery, consciousness, the negative affects* (Vol. 2). New York: Springer.

Toombs, K. (Ed.). (2001). *Handbook of phenomenology and medicine*. Dordrecht: Kluwer Academic Publishers.

van Deurzen, E., & Kenward, R. (2005). *Dictionary of existential psychotherapy and counseling*. London: Sage Publications.

Chapter 6
Health and Illness and Holistic Health

The noun "patient" comes from the Latin *patiens* which means "one who suffers". The adjective also means being able to wait, in the sense of enduring a difficult time. Combining the two concepts, a patient is one who endures suffering. Suffering is a part of the human condition which has always been with us. However, our views on suffering have differed over time and from culture to culture. I will in this chapter look at different conceptions of health and illness[1] in order to prepare the ground for a discussion of what can be meant by a modern conception of "holistic health." The term is often found in the literature, but what is actually meant by holistic health is rarely explicated in a satisfactory way. I will later in this chapter show how the phenomenological theory proposed in this book constitutes a good starting point for a genuinely holistic conception of health.

Various models of health and illness emphasize different aspects of human life. Some theories focus upon health, while others are concerned mainly with sickness and symptoms. Ancient models of health and illness can be characterized as *health* models, as health was considered the natural condition and sickness was something unnatural, often conceived of in terms of punishment from God. The cure was to get back in line with God's will and stay there (Tamm 1994). Sickness and suffering were taken for granted as a part of life and not questioned as such, but the *reason* for suffering was a matter of religious interest. The Jewish-Christian model from the Old and New Testament understood illness as punishment for sins, although Jewish theology was concerned with the distribution of suffering (for example Job), while Christianity became a religion about the vindication of suffering through the Cross.[2] The connection between health and right living is a theme running throughout the history of medicine up to the modern time, although today its importance has been overshadowed by a materialistic view of ill health, which I will return to shortly.

Traditional Western thinking about health and illness has its roots in Ancient Greece, dating back to Hippocrates (460–377 BC), known as the father of Western

---

[1] For the sake of simplicity I will speak of illness as the opposite of health. The term "disease" is too limited as it designates only those conditions with a known diagnosis. Illness refers to the subjective experience of not being well, which is the condition I am interested in explicating.

[2] See Bowker (1970).

J. Bullington, *The Expression of the Psychosomatic Body from a Phenomenological Perspective*, SpringerBriefs in Philosophy,
DOI: 10.1007/978-94-007-6498-9_6,

medicine. Hippocrates showed a surprisingly modern view as he is quoted as saying, "It is more important to know what sort of person has a disease than to know what sort of disease a person has".[3] Around the same period Plato (427–347 BC) wrote, "The cure of many diseases is unknown to the physicians of Hellas, because they disregard the whole which ought to be studied, for the part can never be well unless the whole is well".[4] The Ancient view of holism in the West was based on the concepts of balance and harmony. The main metaphors for describing a healthy human being from this time were; balance between different body fluids (black bile, yellow bile, phlegm and blood), balance between different earthly elements and the body, or balance between the body and the soul. Plato defined health as a state of harmony, equilibrium and order, mimicking the natural order of the Cosmos. One can actually find two tendencies in the ancient Greek view of health and illness, the one which focused on health, the so-called *"Hygiea-principle"*, and the other so-called *"Asklepios-principle"*, which was concerned with treating and curing ill health. *Hygiea* was the Greek Goddess who watched over the health of the people of Athens. She symbolized the healthy human being as *mens sana in corpora sano* (a sound mind in a sound body). *Asklepios* was a legendary doctor who cured people with the knife and medical herbs. The ancient principles of *Hygiea* (prevention) and *Asklepios* (cure) represent two aspects of medicine which are still with us today (Dubos 1959).

The ancient Chinese model of health, so-called "traditional Chinese medicine" (TCM), can also be characterized as a health model, with much attention paid to the prevention of ill health. The emphasis here is also on balance, in this case, balance between the forces of Yin and Yang,[5] balance between an individual/or group and their ancestors, and balance between man and nature. According to this model, it is equally important for one's health how one greets one's neighbor as how one eats or sleeps. The concept of *Qi*, or power of life, is said to play an important role in maintaining health. *Qi*, also meaning "vapor", "steam", or "uncooked rice", is the underlying thread that runs through all of life, flowing constantly between the opposites of Yin and Yang. In human beings, the balance of Yin and Yang is said to be responsible for the health or illness of the person, although there is no absolute standard of which "balance" of Yin and Yang constitutes health. What constitutes sickness for one person may be health for another (Kaptchuk 2000). Both ancient Greek thinking and traditional Chinese medicine include a variety of dimensions as relevant for health which are not intuitively a part of the modern understanding. Living a virtuous life, being in balance with the powers of the Cosmos (Yin and Yang), taking care of one's obligations, these sorts of considerations are seldom associated with health in the

---

3 Hippocrates. http://www.brainyquote.com/quotes/authors/h/hippocrates.html.

4 Plato "Charmides" in *Plato, Collected Dialogues* (1961) s. 103.

5 Yin and Yang are usually characterized as complementary opposites that are inextricably bound up with each other, like for example, night and day, light and dark, masculine and feminine, hot and cold. Originally, the terms referred to the light and dark side of a mountain, exemplifying the ever flowing movement of Yin into Yang and Yang into Yin (moving opposites) as the light, sunny side of the mountain side gradually becomes the dark side as the sun moves during the day.

traditional modern view. In this sense, one could say that the "life- world" of the patient (as we would call it today) has disappeared, as the objective body became the focus of medicine. How did this reductionism come about?

The first real significant medical discovery occurred in 1682, when William Harvey described the circulatory system of the blood stream in the body. Later on, in the middle of the 1800s Rudolf Virchow started to use the concept of the "cell". As scientists learned more about the inner workings of the body, it became common to characterize diseases in terms of structural changes at the cellular level. Another major figure in medicine from the 1800s was Louis Pasteur, who discovered that certain diseases were caused by special microorganisms. Modern medicine rests upon these discoveries, and for that reason, Western medicine can be characterized as a "sickness/disease" model, where the focus is placed upon understanding the mechanisms of disease in biological, material terms (Tamm 1994). According to this model, one is healthy when one is free from disease and no real attention is paid to the condition of health.[6] Ill health (disease) was simply understood as organic processes affecting the body through materialistic causality. These pathological processes could be observed neutrally, independently of culture, moral or societal factors. Classical biomedicine is a reductionistic model, since it reduces health and illness to the materiality of the body. Jewson (1975) pointed out that the more doctors learned about how the body worked, the less interested they became in the lives of their patients.

It is only during the last few hundred years that health has been understood mainly in terms of objectively identifiable processes occurring in the physical body. Throughout history, health has been associated with the notion of balance and harmony, virtue and a moral life, societal norms and behavior. Interestingly enough, the notion of health as balance and harmony can be found in many different cultures throughout different epochs. In ancient Western thinking, "balance" referred to living in harmony with nature (the Gods), with one's fellow human beings, and possessing an inner harmony within oneself, usually characterized as a calm, steady spirit, without violent, uncontrolled emotions. In TCM, the imbalance between Yin and Yang and problems with the flow of Qi in the body are considered to be the main causes of ill health. The intuition that balance has something to do with health is also found in modern theories of health, both lay and professional, as we shall see in the following section.

Modern Theories of Health

The most famous and most often quoted modern definition of health comes from The World Health Organization (WHO), which stated that "Health is a state of

---

[6] This does not mean that people were not concerned with maintaining health. It was simply not the domain of medicine proper. Folk medicine (indigenous medicine, alternative medicine) has always existed side by side with the medical sciences.

complete physical, mental and social well-being and not merely the absence of disease or infirmity" (WHO 1948). Although this definition has been criticized for being utopian, it was important, since it brought social and psychological factors back into the health equation. The reductionistic view of health that had dominated medicine was challenged by a definition that included non-medical aspects of people's lives. This could be said to be the beginning of a more "holistic" view of health and illness in the modern era. A few decades later, the sociologist Claudine Herzlich (1973) performed a well-known study where she asked lay people about their understanding of health and found three groups, which she called "health-in-a-vacuum", "reserve of health" and "equilibrium". The first group described health as not having disease or infirmity, the second group meant that being healthy had to do with being strong in order to withstand fatigue and sickness, while the third, which was the most frequent description found, characterized health as physical well-being, strength, absence of fatigue, psychological well-being, calmness, mobility, effectiveness and good relations to others. It is interesting that these lay perceptions of health reflected both the reductionistic definition of health which WHO had dismissed as inadequate (the absence of disease or infirmity), as well as a description which reminds us of the ancient conceptions of balance and harmony. Indeed, Herzlich named this last category "equilibrium." These findings illustrate how multi-faceted the concept of health can be. In fact, different and sometimes even contradictory notions of a concept can exist peacefully side by side in what Ludwik Fleck (1979) called "thought collectives". Cultural notions are constantly being transformed, negotiated and re-negotiated. In any case, the materialistic, short-lived, reductionistic view of health as the absence of disease eventually had to make room for alternative notions that included non-medical (physical) aspects of life.

The sociologist Talcott Parsons' (1981) writings have also played a part in the modern conception of health and illness. He defined health as a person's ability to fulfill the duties and obligations which are placed upon them according to their existing social position. If the person can no longer live up to the social contract, he or she will be able to take on the "sick-role", sanctioned by society. That is to say, if s/he meets certain criteria, the person will be excused from their social obligations until that time when they are once again capable of resuming their role in society. An important part of the sick-role is the willingness on the part of the sick person to cure/rehabilitate themselves as quickly as possible, in order to show solidarity towards the society supporting them while they (temporarily) cannot perform their societal function. Parsons' theory has been criticized as being too narrow, in that it did not critically examine society. Critics meant that perhaps it is precisely the demands of the society which make people sick.[7] Another trend in modern theories of health is to highlight the importance of personal character attributes such as strength or coping abilities. The medical doctor Oliver Sacks (2001) has the idea

[7] See for example the anti-psychiatry movement in the 1960s with writers such as R. D. Laing, Michel Foucault and Thomas Szasz.

that health has to do with an unwavering metaphysical strength, a "resilient spirit", such as he was able to witness in his clinical work with persons with neurological disorders. Sociologist Rory Williams (1983) had a similar idea about health as a reserve of strength which could be mobilized when needed. Another interesting theme in the literature is that health is the ability to adjust to changing states of affairs.[8] Adaptability seems to play an important role in the ability to sustain health, according to these theories. On a similar note, the so-called "equilibrium theories of health" presented by the Scandinavian philosophers Pörn (1993) and Nordenfelt (1987) define health in terms of successful *interaction* with the environment. Nordenfelt maintains that a person is in health if the person is able to achieve his/her "vital goals" in standard circumstances. He explicitly challenges the bio-statistical theory of health (Boorse 1977), which defines health as the absence of disease, where disease is understood as statistical deviations from a set of measured normal standards. The critique of the bio-statistical model here is the same as against all reductionistic models, namely, we may find persons who should be defined as "unhealthy" who feel absolutely fine, and conversely, people with no measurable deviation from the norm who nevertheless are in obvious ill health. All dimensions of health and illness cannot be measured, and deviations from measured norms are never exclusively responsible for either health or illness. According to the equilibrium theories of health, health can be seen as a balance between an individual's ambitions and goals, life circumstances and competence. Finally, Seedhouse (2001) formulates a definition of health rather like the Scandinavian model, where health is equivalent to the state of conditions which enables persons to work in order to fulfill realistic choices and biological potentials, health is thus the "foundation for achievement". The degree of health in this model depends upon how well the person is able to realize their potential.

So, most modern theories describe health as a form of successful interaction between man's abilities, values, goals and life circumstances and his/her environment. This is surprisingly similar to the ancient thinking as well as the phenomenological theory of psychosomatics presented in the previous chapter. It is now time to approach the question of "holistic health" What can this term mean?

Holistic Health

As illustrated above, health has been understood as the absence of disease only during a relatively short period of history. A more complex conception of health has historical roots in notions about balance and harmony, virtue and morality, societal norms and behavior, in short, a good life. Modern health theories are an attempt to break the reductionistic dominance of the disease model and bring the sick *person* back onto the scene. A modern, holistic understanding of health

[8] See Mansfield (1977), Dubos (1959) and Illich (1977).

includes biological, psychological and social factors as well as highlights the importance of how individuals are able to successfully interact with their environment. The choices people make and the opportunities they are given (or not given) are also relevant for understanding health. This means that things like autonomy, choice and quality of life become important for defining health (Seedhouse 2001). So according to this picture of holism, it is not enough to include the psycho-social aspects of an individual's life in order to have a holistic theory, one must also take into account the way in which the individual interacts (successfully or unsuccessfully) with their environment. With this in mind, let us now examine how "holistic health"/"holistic care" is reflected in the scientific literature.

The term "holism" was first introduced into academic texts by a philosopher named Jan Christian Smuts who wrote about holism in connection to chemistry (1926). His definition of holism was that the sum was greater than the parts, an idea also found in Gestalt psychology of the 20s and 30s. Nursing science especially became influenced by the concept of holism during the 70s and it has been a prominent feature of nursing theory ever since (McEvoy and Duffy 2008), even if there are some dissenting voices.[9] A search on the Internet for scientific articles on "holistic care" "holistic medicine" and "holistic treatment" yields thousands of hits, including articles on alternative/complementary treatment methods as well as those studies which claim to have a biological-psychological-social approach to health care problems. I will in the following presentation exclude literature on alternative/complementary medicine and focus on articles which purport to use or clarify a "holistic" approach. There have been a number of theoretical attempts to define what "holistic care" means (Berg and Sarvimäki 2003; Bush and Bruni 2008; McEvoy and Duffy 2008) as well as a variety of empirical studies purporting to use a "holistic" framework in clinical practice (Borwick 2011; Brown and Wimpenny 2011; Henderson 2002; Hjelm et al. 2003; Odey 2009; Zengerle-Levy 2004).[10] The term "holistic" functions most often in these texts as a negative category, that is, as a name for that which is *not* reductionistic medicine. For example, holistic care is characterized as non-technical, non-task oriented (relation-oriented), non-fragmented, non-utilitarian, non-statistical and so on. The term is introduced as an alternative to the strictly medical approach, although what it actually entails is not clearly defined. The "whole" in holism is the idea that the whole (the human being) is more than the sum of the parts, an implicit (sometimes explicit) criticism of the biomedical tradition that only tends to the somatic "part" of the human being. Proponents of holistic care and holistic health are attentive to individual, emotional, social, psychological, existential (and sometimes spiritual)

---

[9] For example, "Holism is a default term employed too often in place of a clearer and more precise language to describe the perspective and unique contribution of nursing". (Reed 2000 p. 131).

[10] Most of this literature comes from nursing science. Holism has become an important hallmark for the nursing profession, distinguishing them from the medical doctors whom they once "served" as biomedical assistants.

dimensions of the human being. One often finds references given to notions of "balance" "harmony" and "whole", but these terms are not defined.[11] There is nothing inherently wrong with this perspective. On the contrary, it is laudable. However, the texts are often riddled by a vagueness and lack of philosophical rigor which gives the entire approach an air of New Age which does not further the cause.[12]

What would a holistic theory of health need in order to gain credibility and influence in the area of the health care sciences? First of all, one would need to clearly define the concepts used and explain how they are relevant for understanding the area under study. Secondly, one would need to explicate the way in which the terms used related to each other. Thirdly, any purported lines of causality or influence (between mind–body–world) would need to be grounded in empirical evidence or theoretical argumentation. Finally, the theory would need to make clear which ontological pre-suppositions are in place and how this ontological position is both reasonable and fruitful for the object of the theory, in this case, holistic health.

In the scientific literature, the terms most often used for defining the holistic approach to health are: the whole person, healing, integration, wellness, balance, holistic assessment, holistic approach and holistic focus.[13] The fact that these terms are used without any explanation in the text can indicate that the authors assume that the reader already shares the ideology of holism, or is at least is skeptical to reductionistic biomedicine. For this reason, the (implicit) shared position of "holism" is does not need to be explained. This is problematic, since exactly what holism entails can mean a variety of things. The theoretical articles that attempt to define holism use either concept analysis or try to synthesize the

---

[11] For example, "Occupational health nurses who create life balance can be fully present for clients" (Riley 2003, p. 439), and "[…] as the nursing profession has traditionally viewed the person as a whole, concerned with the interrelationship of body, mind and spirit […]" (McEvoy and Duffy 2008, p. 414) and "A wholistic approach in nursing […] implies a view of man as being a whole, consisting of a physical, psychological social and spiritual dimension." (Berg and Sarvimäki 2003, p. 384.) One would like to know, what is "life balance"? How do the authors conceive of the "interrelationship" between body, mind and spirit? In what way is the "whole" constituted by physical, psychological and social "dimensions"? That which is missing here is a conceptual, philosophical grounding of the terms and a proper explication of the proposed interrelations between them.

[12] There are some exceptions (Reed 2000; Strandberg et al. 2007; Thorn 2001) where the focus is a critical, analytic approach to the use of these terms.

[13] For example: "Holistic self care attends to the needs of the *whole* person and although the effects of body, mind and spirit cannot be separated from the whole, bringing attention to each component can help nurses set the intention to care for their whole selves" (Riley 2003, p. 439) and […] the goal of achieving *balance across domains of wellness* is seen as a lifelong process […] (Gieck and Olsen 2007, p. 30) and "Although nursing aims to treat the "*whole person*", sexuality and sexual health are not always seen as an integral part of the whole person." (Odey 2009, p. 43) and "After performing a *holistic assessment* of a patient's needs […] (Borwick 2011, p. 36) and "Appropriate *holistic assessment* seems vital in provision of care to the obese individual" (Brown and Wimpenny 2011, p. 10) my emphasis in italics.

various meanings in order to construct a working definition of "holistic care". Some writers simply draw the conclusion that holism is not a viable concept and should be abandoned in favor of more precise terminology.

On the matter of how the various concepts involved in a holistic theory relate to each other there is no explicit argumentation. There may be "balancing, interacting and competing influences of the mind, body, environment and spirit" (Hjelm et al. 2003, p. 353) or "[...] a living nexus between spiritual care, spirituality and holism" (Bush and Bruni 2008, p. 539) but as long as these descriptions are not adequately explicated they are of little use. Neither does one find any explicit discussion of causality (how mind, body, sprit and world interact) in the literature, nor specific ontological statements, other than very general ones, often with references to phenomenological or existentialist philosophers. To focus on patients' experiences is not wrong, but for a holistic theory of health to gain status in the scientific community, we need more than declamations that one is interested in the "life-world" of the patient.

However, if the empirical scientific literature is weak with regards to explicating how the lived body and the concept of the life-world enhance our understanding of health care issues, there are a variety of sound texts from the disciplines of philosophy (Al-Saji 2008; Carel 2008; Johnson 1987; Gallagher 1995, 2005; Leder 1990; Tolero 2005; Toombs, 1995, 2001), sociology (Turner 2001; Williams and Bendelow 1998), anthropology (Csordas 1994; Desjarlais and Throop 2011; Knibbe and Versteeg 2008), caring sciences (Benner 1994, 2001; Dahlberg et al. 2007), women's studies (Ahmed 2007; Jacobson 2011; Young 2005) and architecture (Pallasmaa 2005) which take up interesting aspects of lived body (a phenomenological perspective on the body) in relation to their specific area of study. These authors often address embodiment issues in a way that could be of interest and inspiration for those who work within the area of health care.

To sum up thus far, we have seen that modern theories of health include not only psycho-social aspects of human life but underscore the significance of how successfully persons are able to interact with his/her environment. The notion of balance is used, as in ancient theories of health, in order to try to capture something intuitively significant about the experience of being in good health. In the modern view, health can be understood as a "harmony" between goals and achievement, between specific ambitions, competence and opportunities. Personal characteristics such as being able to adapt to new situations, having a resilient spirit and a reserve of strength are said to play a role in maintaining health. One could characterize these modern theories as holistic (in the sense of addressing more than one "part" of the human being), although mind–body-world interaction is assumed here rather than subjected to philosophical scrutiny, as the theoreticians are not specifically interested this philosophical issue per se. We have also seen above that although "holistic health" and "holistic care" are frequently used in the scientific literature, these terms seem to function more as ideological positioning *against* biomedicine than a philosophically grounded alternative to reductionism. Let me now turn to my own phenomenological theory and see how it fares in relation to the criteria of clear terminology, comprehensible causation and clearly stated ontological pre-suppositions. Afterwards, I will discuss how this theory provides a reasonable ground for many of our lay and professional (theoretical) intuitions about health as balance and successful interaction with the environment. In this way, a holistic theory of health can gain philosophical clarity and credibility.

Holistic Health in Terms of the Phenomenological Theory of Psychosomatics

The terminology used in the phenomenological theory of psychosomatics comes from the philosophical work of Merleau-Ponty. The relevant terms in this theory are: the lived body, structure transformation, the "dialogue" between man and world, meaning and expression, reversibility and the flesh. The explication of these terms has been laid out extensively in Chaps. 2–4, so, as to the issue of clearly defined terminology, the theory clearly meets the above mentioned criterion. The question of how these terms relate to each other (the actual *theory* of psychosomatics) is the topic of Chap. 5. In terms of ontological pre-suppositions, the strategic choice of using Merleau-Ponty's phenomenology as the philosophical starting point for the theory is motivated by the need to bypass the dead ends presented by classical dualism and materialistic reductionism outlined in Chap. 1. Because I do not begin with a dualistic or reductionsitic framework, I will not have to worry about how mind and body can interact (dualism), or explain how a psychosomatic condition can arise if there is no psychosocial reality (materialism). There is no mystery about a "speaking body" when we understand that the body is capable of expression as *lived* body. For this reason, the phenomenology of Merleau-Ponty is decidedly a relevant and fruitful starting for understanding health and illness as ways of being-in-the-world. However, the issue of etiology (causation) is something I would like to address briefly here, since the phenomenological perspective is quite different from the everyday, natural attitude and must therefore be constantly clarified in order to avoid misunderstandings.

The word "etiology" comes from the Greek *aitiologia,* the root *aitia* meaning "guilt" in the sense of owing someone something. The Latin term *causa* was originally a legal term, having to do with questions of liability. Thus, in its etymological sense, "cause" connotes something bad, or at least something out of the ordinary. On-going, normal events are seldom candidates for causes, although they do form the background context within which a cause may effectuate an event, like the way the presence of oxygen allows the match to ignite. In the natural sciences, causes are observable, verifiable processes or chains of events happening in the material world, most often referring to unusual, out-of-the-ordinary things. In the case of illness, biomedicine looks for signs of material processes (at various levels of the body) which are said to be responsible (*causa*) for the ill health.[14] The objective body admits of this level of causation, for example, a virus *causes* a the flu, a broken arm *cause*s pain, a stroke *causes* paralysis etc. but the lived body of the subject (the mind–body-world unity of the flesh) is not amenable to the type of causation found in the natural sciences. A particular problem is that it is difficult to discuss etiology in any other terms than those of the objective body, since we have learned to look at ill health precisely as objective, on-going physiological processes in a material body. As soon as we start to speak of "tumors", "headaches" and "back pains", we find ourselves automatically within the perspective of the objective body, and visualize before us certain physiological processes taking place in an impersonal, objective body. This is natural for us, since we have learned what a tumor *is* from within the perspective of the objective body. So the question is, how can we maintain our focus on the lived body and at the same time discuss the "etiology" of conditions which we have learned to think about in terms of impersonal, third-person processes going on in the material body?

The first thing we need to do is remind ourselves of what ill health *is* according to the phenomenological theory of psychosomatics. It is not the causal result of material processes in the body, but first and foremost the breakdown of meaning-constitution at the proper (psycho-social) level, resulting in a disarticulated field (the world pole of the lived body) and the stagnation of the subject-world dialogue. No structure transformations occur and the body meaning (the inarticulate signaling of the symptom) becomes the only "answer" to the problematic life situation. With this in mind, the question of the "cause" of the experience of illness must be found in the lived, "in-between" experience of the persons' relationship to their world. This is not to say that the objective, material body plays no role in bad health, it is merely to point out that the phenomenological theory presented in this book does not attribute bad health to material processes in the body, but rather, focuses upon how the body, self and world are *lived* in the chiasm which is human experience.[15] This perspective solves the paradox that certain persons we would

[14] This perspective is the guiding principle behind so-called "evidence based medicine" (EBM), which has been both praised and criticized during the last 20 years. "Evidence" within this paradigm for choosing either the one or the other medical intervention is comprised of large samples of empirical, randomized control (trail) studies (so-called "RCT studies"). The kind of knowledge that can be generated by this type of study is said to be the "golden standard" for scientific knowledge to be used in medicine, and if knowledge cannot be validated in this way, it is not considered to be scientifically interesting. Although the original idea behind evidence based medicine was to take into account not only experimental studies but also the experience of the practitioner and the patient's point of view, evidence based medicine has, for many, become synonymous with the positivistic view of knowledge which claims that only that which can be operationalized, measured and validated experimentally constitutes true knowledge.

[15] Merleau-Ponty writes: "Tiredness does not halt my companion, because he likes to feel himself in the midst of things, to feel their rays converging upon him [...] my own fatigue brings me to a halt because I dislike it, because I have chosen differently in my manner of being in the world, because, for instance, I endeavor, not to be in nature, but rather to win the recognition of others" (1945/1962, p. 441).

call "ill" claim to be in good health, while others with no material signs of symptoms are indeed in very bad health. The phenomenological focus on the mind–body-world system (rather than the "somatic" part) is a different perspective which we must constantly remind ourselves in order to avoid falling back into the causal etiology of biomedicine. So the answer to the question of etiology is not to isolate physiology, juxtapose upon it a psychological level and hope that no one notices the incompatibility of these terms (the classical problem within psychosomatic theory described in Chap. 1). The answer is to find a third term wherein we can understand both physiology and psychology simultaneously as the ambiguous, intertwined, embodied subjectivity of existence. The etiology of psychosomatic symptoms refers not to the interaction of a consciousness with the "stuff" of the material body, but to the integrated way in which the subject "chooses" to express his/her difficulties at the level of the body, resulting in the specific psychosomatic way of being-in-the-world described in Chap. 5.

The next question is, can this theory, designed to help us understand psychosomatic pathology, aid in understanding what "holistic health" could be? Let us first recapitulate what modern theories of health bring to the table, and then return to the difficulties outlined above in connection to the scientific literature on holistic health. First of all, holistic theories of health focus upon the *person*, with his/her psychosocial reality, challenging the reductionistic view of health as the absence of disease, understood in terms of the material body. The notion of "balance" is often invoked in these theories, in some form (equilibrium, balance etc.), although the concept is not defined nor discussed in the literature. Modern theories of health focus on individual character attributes (such as having a resilient spirit and adaptability) and the importance of successful interaction with the environment for the experience of health. Many of these insights are actually modern reformulations of ancient notions which have been with us for thousands of years, both in Western and Eastern systems of thought. The most serious problems connected to the scientific literature addressing "holistic health" is the vagueness of the terminology and the non-explicated links or lines of influence between subjective experiences of health and the various multi-factors said to be involved in health and illness. This is where the phenomenological theory can provide proper clarification and explication on these issues.

Let us begin with the terminology used in holistic health literature, especially the term "the whole person". Although this undefined term is used mainly as a critique of biomedicine which only addresses a "part" of the whole, we can agree that a holistic theory of health and health care must try to fulfill WHO's definition of health, and in some way take into account the psychosocial well being of the person. Merleau-Ponty's notion of the lived body, as the total system of the mind–body-world unity, is a good description of this whole, as it focuses upon the way in which the person (as a mind–body unity) attends to the presence of the world, as it shows itself to that person in the particular, lived situation. The lived body is a description of the "whole", although in order to properly understand what is being described, one must leave the natural attitude and enter the phenomenological perspective. The concept of the lived body maintains the reality of the psychosocial realm of existence (against materialistic reductionism) but also introduces the idea of meaning-constitution at the level of the body. Furthermore, the lived body also includes the world, as a lived situation, thus providing in these three "poles" of the lived body a holistic description of mind–body and world (the "environment"-as-lived by the subject). The writings of Merleau-Ponty also address the interaction between man (as a mind–body unity) and world in terms of clearly articulated concepts, such as the intentional arc, motor intentionality, expression, reversibility and the chiasm. In this way, the concept of the lived body (and the later notion of the flesh) provide a fully developed account of mind, body and world as well as addressing the issue of "interaction" between them.

Further terms in need of clarification for a holistic theory of health are "balance" "integration" "equilibrium" and the like. The literature is full of these concepts although they are not explicated. I propose that the notion of structure transformation and "harmony-of-situation" described in the phenomenological theory may provide these terms with a suitable content. As described in Chap. 5, when a situation can be responded to through meaning-constitution at the proper level, we find "harmony" and "balance" in the sense that there is no tension or unresolved "gestalt" in need of structure transformation. The proper level (on the mind–body continuum) of meaning constitution has been achieved, either through habitual sedimentation (if the situation is familiar) or through structure transformations, if the person needs to modify his/her structures in order to accommodate the new situation, in the latter case creating fresh new meanings and horizons to be explored. The advantage of understanding balance in terms of structure transformations is that is gives us a way to conceptualize the "meeting" between man and situation. When we understand meaning as the lived intertwining (chiasm) between man and situation, we can investigate the orientation of the subject towards the world and see where meaning-constitution has broken down. That state referred to as an unspecified "equilibrium" in the literature can now be explicated as the harmony-of-situation in the lived body. One does not have to go as far as the formation of psychosomatic symptoms in order to make use of this understanding of harmony and balance. The lack of well-being related to illness has to do with having one's being-in-the-world disrupted, to a greater or lesser degree. The degree of disruption will correspond to what extent the health problem (broken leg, diabetes, migraine, lumbago, etc.) interferes with one's goals, sense of self and perception of the world (the "environment" with which one interacts). According to this view of health, one can be in more or less good health even if one has a disease and conversely, experience ill health even if there is no corresponding objective sign (physical processes causing symptoms) in the physical body.

There is an intuitive understanding in modern health theories that the ability to adapt to various life situations is important for being able to maintain health. Adaptability can also be understood in terms of the ability to transform and sediment structures in order to expand the range of experiences of oneself and the world. The more of the world that one can "see" and experience, the more one can realize the human drive towards transcendence, which is characteristic for our way of being-in-the-world. Both self and world are involved in the movement of becoming, and as long as one can "adapt" in this process, one experiences health. Adaption, in this sense, is a term that describes adequate structure transformation. Non-adaption, or unsuccessful adaption, would be when structure transformation is not possible and the person's habitual, sedimented way of experiencing and understanding the world does not fit the situation. It is clear that the easier one has adapting to the new, the greater the chances that one will be equipped to meet a variety of life challenges, thus minimizing the risk for long-term stress reactions and psychosomatic symptoms. Another idea found in modern holistic health theories is that health has to do with achieving goals and realizing possibilities in line with ones' values and capabilities. The achievement of vital goals is certainly involved in the experience of health, and can be understood as the way in which human beings strive towards more and more nuanced articulation of self and world. As creatures of language, culture and social life, we find ourselves in a world which is given to us as the place where we are to live our lives and achieve our goals. To the extent to which we are successful in realizing our goals (through interacting with our environment), we will experience ourselves as more or less competent and adult, more or less successful in articulating a self in terms of our values, ambitions and desires. In line with this, a phenomenological definition of health, according to the theory outlined in this book, would be that health is that way of being-in-the-world wherein a variety of situations can arise, be sustained and develop in the continual unfolding of meaning-constitution, where both subject and meaningful world (successful structure transformation) evolve over time.

Because this theory provides a non-dualistic, non-reductionistic framework, it is ideal for articulating a holistic theory of health. Although the theory is designed to specifically address psychosomatic ill health, it is possible to incorporate the theory into any type of holistic health assessment. For example, if a young man has broken his arm, a strictly biomedical approach would be to take care of the fracture (a cast and a sling), see to it that he is informed as to how to take care of his fracture and perhaps subscribe some pain medication. A holistic view would attend to other dimensions than the material, such as, what does it *mean* for this individual at this point in time to not have the use of his arm? He may be, for example, trying out for the baseball team at school, and lose precious training time when he can't practice. His home situation may be such that his parents are putting pressure on him to excel in sports. He may imagine that the only way to attract the attention of the girls he is interested in is to become a baseball star at school. One of his "vital goals" is therefore to make the baseball team. This means that a simple fracture may not be so simple for this boy, and health care professionals need to attend to this, if we want to say that we are really seeing "the whole" person. Using the insights of the lived body, it may even be so that the boy's identity, intentional arc, dialogue with his world and his ability to sustain various situations (like studying) also suffer during this time, resulting in an ill health that does not primarily have to do with his fracture, but more with how this fracture is lived and how it transforms his view of himself and what the world can "afford" him in terms of possible situations, when he has his arm in a cast.

So, when we speak about holistic health and holistic assessment, it is necessary fill the terms with a content that gives us tools we can use to understand health in terms of WHOs "[...] mental and social well-being and not merely the absence of disease or infirmity". The phenomenological theory outlined in this book fulfills the criteria needed in order to ground "holistic health" in a philosophical framework. In the following final chapter, I will examine what this view of health and illness means for the clinical praxis of health care.

References

Ahmed, S. (2007). *Queer phenomenology: orientations, objects, others*. Durham and London: Duke University Press.

Al-Saji, A. (2008). A past which has never been present: Bergsonian dimensions in Merleau-Ponty's theory of the prepersonal. *Research in Phenomenology, 38*, 41–71.

Benner, P. (1994). The tradition and skill of interpretative phenomenology in studying health, illness and caring practices. In P. Benner (Ed.), *Interpretive phenomenology: embodiment, caring and ethics in health and illness*. Thousand Oaks: Sage Publications Ltd.

Benner, P. (2001). The phenomenon of care. In K. Toombs (Ed.), *Handbook of Phenomenology and medicine*. Dordrecht: Kluwer Academic Publishers.

Berg, G. V., & Sarvimäki, A. (2003). A holistic-existential approach to health promotion. *Scandinavian Journal of Caring Science, 17*, 384–391.

Boorse, C. (1977). Health as a theoretical concept. *Philosophy of Science, 44*, 542–573.

Borwick, G. (2011). A holistic approach to meeting the needs of patients with conditions that affect their appearance. *Primary Health Care, 21*(1), 33–39.

Bowker, J. (1970). *Problems of suffering in religions of the World*. Cambridge: Cambridge University Press.

Brown, J., & Wimpenny, P. (2011). Developing a holistic approach to obesity management. *International Journal of Nursing Practice, 17*, 9–18.

Bush, T., & Bruni, N. (2008). Spiritual care as a dimension of holistic care: a relational interpretation. *International Journal of Palliative Nursing, 14*(11), 539–545.

Carel, H. (2008). *Illness*. Stocksfield: Acumen.

T. Csordas (Ed.), (1994). *Embodiment and experience: The existential ground of culture and self.* Cambridge: Cambridge University Press.

Dahlberg, K., Nyström, M., & Dahlberg, H. (2007). *Reflective lifeworld research*. Lund: Studentlitteratur.

Desjarlais, R., & Throop, J. C. (2011). Phenomenological approaches in anthropology. *Annual Review of Anthropology, 40*, 87–102.

Dubos, R. (1959). *The mirage of health*. New York: Harper and Row.

Fleck, L. (1979). *The genesis and development of a scientific fact*. Chicago: University of Chicago Press.

Gallagher, S. (1995). Body schema and intentionality. In J.A. Bermúdez, A. Marcel/N. Elian (Eds.), *The Body and the Self.* Cambridge: The MIT press.

Gallagher, S. (2005). *How the body shapes the mind*. Oxford: Clarendon Press.

Gieck, J. D., & Olsen, S. (2007). Holistic wellness as a means to developing a lifestyle approach to health behavior among college students. *Journal of American College Health, 56*(1), 29–35.

Henderson, S. (2002). Factors impacting on nurses' transference of theoretical knowledge of holistic care into clinical practice. *Nurse Education in Practice, 2*, 244–250.

Herzlich, C. (1973). *Health and illness: a social psychological analysis*. London: Academic Press.

Hippocrates. http://www.brainyquote.com/quotes/authors/h/hippocrates.html

Hjelm, K., Rolfe, M., Bryar, R. M., Andersson, B.-L., & Fletcher, M. (2003). Holism in community leg ulcer management: A comparison of nurses in Sweden and the UK. *British Journal of Community Nursing, 8*(8), 353–363.

Illich, I. (1977). *The limits of medicine*. London: Pelican books.

Jacobson, K. (2011). Embodied domestics, embodied politics: Women, home, and agoraphobia. *Human Studies, 34*, 1–21.

Jewson, N. D. (1975). The Disappearance of the Sick Man from Medical Cosmology, 1770–1870. *Sociology, 10*(2), 225–244.

Johnson, M. (1987). *The body in the mind: The bodily basis of meaning, imagination, and reason*. Chicago and London: The University of Chicago Press.

Kaptchuk, T. J. (2000). *The web that has no weaver*. New York: Contemporary Books Inc.

Knibbe, K., & Versteeg, P. (2008). Assessing phenomenology in anthropology: lessons from the study of religion and experience. *Critique of Anthropology, 28*(47), 47–62.

Leder, D. (1990). *The absent body*. Chicago: The University of Chicago Press.

Mansfield, K. (1977). *Letters and journals*. London: Pelican Books.

McEvoy, L., & Duffy, A. (2008). Holistic practice—a conceptual analysis. *Nurse Education in Practice, 8*, 412–419.

Merleau-Ponty, M. (1945/1962). *Phenomenology of Perception*. London: Routledge & Kegan Paul.

Nordenfelt, Lennart. (1987). *On the nature of health: An action-theoretic approach*. Dordrecht: Reidel Publishing.

Odey, K. (2009). Legitimizing patient sexuality and sexual health to provide holistic care. *Gastrointestinal Nursing, 7*(8), 43–47.

Pallasmaa, J. (2005). The eyes of the skin: Architecture and the senses. John Wiley & Sons, UK.

Parsons, T. (1981). Definitions of health and illness in the light of American values and social structure. In A. L. Caplan, H. T. Englehardt Jr, & J. J. McCartney (Eds.), *Concepts of health and disease Interdisciplinary Perspectives*. USA: Addison-Wesley Publishing.

Plato (1961). *Charmides in Plato, Collected Dialogues*. New Jersey: Princeton University Press.

Pörn, I. (1993). Health and adaptedness. *Theoretical Medicine, 14*, 295–303.

Reed, P. G. (2000). Nursing reformation: Historical reflections and philosophic foundations. *Nursing Science Quarterly, 13*(2), 129–136.

Riley, J. B. (2003). Holistic self care: Strategies for initiating a personal assessment. *AAOHJ Journal, 51*(10), 439–447.

Sacks, O. (2001). *Awakenings*. New York: Harper Perennial.

Seedhouse, D. (2001). *Health: the foundations for achievement*. New York: John Wiley & Sons Ltd.

Smuts, J. C. (1926). *Holism and evolution*. New York: Macmillan.

Strandberg, E. L., Ovhed, I., Borgqvist, L., & Wilhelmsson, S. (2007). The perceived meaning of a (w)holistic view among general practitioners and district nurses in Swedish primary care: a qualitative study. *BMC Family Practice,*8:8. doi:10.1186/1471-2296/8/8.

Tamm, M. (1994). *Modeller för hälsa och sjukdom*. Malmö: Tiger Förlag.

Thorn, S. E. (2001). People and their parts: Deconstructing the debates in theorizing nursing's clients. *Nursing Philosophy, 2*, 259–262.

Tolero, M. (2005). Perception, normativity, and Selfhood in Merleau-Ponty: the spatial level and existential space. *The Southern Journal of Philosophy, 43*, 443–461.

Toombs, K. (Ed.) (1995). *Chronic illness: From experience to policy*. Indiana: Indiana University Press.

Toombs, K. (Ed.). (2001). *Handbook of phenomenology and medicine*. Dordrecht: Kluwer Academic Publishers.

Turner, B. S. (2001). Disability and the sociology of the body. In G. L. Albrecht, K. D. Seelman, & M. Bury (Eds.), *Handbook of disability studies* (pp. 252–266). Thousand Oaks: Sage Publication Inc.

Williams, R. (1983). Concepts of health: an analysis of lay logic. *Sociology, 17*(2), 185–205.

Williams, S., & Bendelow, G. (1998). *The lived body: sociological themes, embodied issues*. London & New York: Routledge.

World Health Organization (1948). Official records of the World Health Organization, 2.
Young, I. M. (2005). *On female body experience: Throwing like a girl and other essays*. Oxford: Oxford University Press.
Zengerle-Levy, K. (2004). Practices that facilitate critically burned Children's holistic healing. *Qualitative Health Research, 14*(9), 1255–1275.

Chapter 7
Conclusions

We have seen in the previous chapters how patients who do not fit into the reductionistic framework with identifiable, material problems in the "machine-body" fall off the grid within traditional health care, since they have neither psychological problems (as they experience their situation) nor somatic problems (as the health care professionals assess their situation). They have problems with their being-in-the-world in the "in-between" which gives both man and world meaning, according to the phenomenological theory offered in this book. In order to grasp this psychosomatic grey zone (neither mind nor body, yet somehow both) we need an alternative theory which takes the mind-body-world unity into account, thereby circumventing the problems associated with dualism and materialistic reductionism. The phenomenological theory of psychosomatics presented in this book grounds an understanding of psychosomatic pathology in a relevant ontology, gives us meaningful concepts to describe and understand this realm of the "in-between", and provides a way to holistically conceptualize health care problems of all kinds, not only psychosomatic ones, by complementing the perspective of the objective body with the lived body.

Patients seeking help for health problems which are not acute often enter the health care system through primary health care. Although "holism" is the word of the day here, many of the solutions offered to persons suffering from ill health are still treatments aimed at the objective body, such as medication and traditional physical therapy. This is all well and good in many cases, but when patients have more complex problems that include psychosocial aspects of life, these purely somatic treatment solutions will not help. If the nature of the health problem is psychosomatic, given the definition in this book, that is, a bodily attempt to solve a problem which demands a solution on a higher level, these patients will wander in the system from doctor to doctor, physical therapist to physical therapist, in a downward spiral which makes it harder to approach the patient with a psychosomatic explanation of their health problems. Finally, the patient will eventually be ejected from the system, since the biomedical repertoire cannot cure these patients' ill health. If the person is referred to a specialized clinic, such as a pain clinic or a psychiatric out-patient center, they may meet a multi-professional team.

J. Bullington, *The Expression of the Psychosomatic Body from a Phenomenological Perspective*, SpringerBriefs in Philosophy,
DOI: 10.1007/978-94-007-6498-9_7, © The Author(s) 2013

If they are lucky, this team will be able to help them relinquish the desire for a somatic solution and begin to work on the patient's problem from a variety of perspectives other than the biomedical one. The question is, does it have to go this far (specialized clinics) in order for persons with these kinds of problems to get adequate help?

It is beyond the scope of this book to give a detailed account of the organization of health care facilities. This may vary from country to country, from rural to urban setting and so on. I will merely give some suggestions for taking care of these patients that can be implemented in a variety of settings without too much organizational or economic difficulty. One strategy is to allow two or more members of staff take a special responsibility for the patients who exhibit psychosomatic, complex health problems. Ideally, representatives from two professions would be involved, such as a psychologist and a nurse, or a physical therapist and a doctor, or an occupational therapist and a nurse/doctor. If the workplace does not have professions other than doctors and nurses, efforts could be made to establish contact with a psychologist or physiotherapist working privately, or within another sector of the health care organization. This pair would meet these patients, individually and/or in group, in order to work on the redefinition phase, that is, help the patient reframe the somatic definition of their problems to a psychosomatic perspective. They would explain the psychosomatic connection and motivate patients to investigate this new line of thinking about their condition. Body work such as body awareness training, grounding exercises, dance and other forms of body expression could be one part of the treatment offered. At the same time, patients would be encouraged to express themselves in terms other than body symptoms. This could be done in individual or group therapy, along the lines given in Chap. 5.

Another strategy for the workplace would be that the entire staff takes part in psychosomatic supervision from a supervisor outside of the workplace with special competence in this area. Through weekly or monthly discussion of psychosomatic cases, the staff would raise the level of competency in the group and be more willing to try different ways of working with these patients. Instead of being provoked by them, the staff could begin to see the group as an interesting clinical challenge, and together work out treatment strategies that would be feasible for their specific workplace. If neither of these options described above are possible, a final recommendation would be to establish contact with persons outside the workplace who have the competence to take these patients into treatment. Building up a network for referral would at least provide the patients somewhere to go when there are no more options left at the level of primary care. A minimum for every workplace coming in contact with patients who have psychosomatic health problems would be to be able to initiate redefinition work, so that patients become motivated to seek adequate help and give up the desire for a purely somatic (biomedical) solution to their ill health.

How can the theory worked out in this book be of use for those patients who do not have psychosomatic problems? As mentioned in Chap. 6, "holistic" health care is a buzz word that needs to be filled with content if it is to be of any use in clinical practice. My suggestion with regards to general health care (that is, not specifically psychosomatic problems) is that all health care professionals should be capable of talking with patients in such a way as to ascertain how the person experiences his/her ill health in his/her way of being-in-the-world, if this is deemed to be of importance for the treatment.[1] This means that every health care professional is aware that the lived body of the patient is a larger perspective than the objective body, and that a different kind of dialogue is needed to bring the lived body into the consulting room. This type of dialogue is not meant to replace the biomedical interrogation of the objective body, but is a complement to it, which can be used when the professional has reason to believe that the patient needs to express how they are affected by or how they experience their situation. It may be that a patient is not complying with the treatment guidelines, or seems unable to cope with their situation, engaging in dangerous or careless acting out behaviors. A patient at an acute ward or a home for the elderly may ring for staff time and time again, asking for things that seem insignificant, irritating the nurses who have a lot to do. A patient may continually bring up an issue that is "outside" of the health problem per se, like a noisy apartment neighbor, a broken car etc., but after a time the health care professional realizes that this needs to be addressed in order to help the patient achieve health. In all of these cases, a special attitude is needed in order to penetrate the significance of the patients "life-world". This attitude can be compared to the phenomenological attitude, where one brackets one's pre-conceived notions and becomes open to that which shows itself, in this case, the way in which the patient constitutes the meaning of their situation.[2] The health care worker implements the phenomenological reduction in order to become truly present to the meaning of what the patient is saying, or needs to express. Let me give some examples from my own teaching of this way of communicating with patients in order to illustrate what kind of dialogue this entails.

When I teach students how to communicate in this way, the first step is to become aware of the way in which one often unconsciously avoids investigating the life world of the patient in the clinical encounter. This pertains to mainly to students who are struggling to integrate their (medical) profession into their way of communicating, but even licensed professionals can have this problem. If one is trained first and foremost in the area of the objective body, it will be these signals that catch one's attention when the patient is speaking. One is trained to listen to descriptions of the objective body, and many of the questions one has in one's repertoire pertain to the machine body, for example, when did you first notice this

[1] This does not mean that every patient needs this form of dialogue. Some patients are perfectly content with the prescription block or the massage. Indeed, they would feel violated if the health care professional started to question them about their experiences of living with ill health. This type of communication should be simply something that one has at ones disposal, in those cases where it is deemed relevant.

[2] This is not really doing phenomenology as the goal is not to ascertain knowledge about phenomena, but rather to gain a deeper understanding of a particular person's situation. But when one knows a bit about phenomenology, one can understand the concept of bracketing.

rash? How long have you had these headaches? How much blood did you lose? What was your insulin count this morning? And so on. This kind of communication we call "fact-gathering" and although such information has its place in a health care encounter, it will not facilitate an atmosphere where the patient feels free to speak about his experiences.[3] The next hinder for the open dialogue about the patients' experiences is the professional's desire to "fix" problems. If a patient says s/he can't sleep, the professional suggests sleeping medications, relaxation techniques or autohypnosis techniques. If the patient is frustrated, one "comforts" them by telling them it will be all right, or that they are doing a great job and so on. These kinds of responses can be first and foremost a matter of soothing the anxiety of the professional and are not always helpful to the patient. The third hurdle is the natural aversion to "meddling" in private matters, which, in this context, is often expressed in terms of students not wanting to feel uncomfortable or to find themselves out of their depths. What if the patient starts to cry, or has a nervous breakdown? When the students have learned that it takes an effort to *not* gather facts, fix problems, give comfort and avoid private topics, they are ready to learn the technique or method, which consists basically of the open (phenomenological) attitude, using questions that "open" rather than "shut" down dialogue, and developing an ear for the *significance* of what is being said in relation to the patient's health problem.

To be "open" in the sense of being present to the patient means that one suspends the natural attitude and puts aside all previous ideas and hypotheses about the way things are. If a patient says "it is so tiresome having small children" we do not automatically assume that we know what she means. We put aside what we think we know about being the mother of small children and ask "in what way is it tiresome for you…?" We take as our starting point that we don't know what this means for her, and we need to ask her to describe her experience, both for herself and for us, in order to get a better grasp of how this situation is being lived. Openness means we are willing to investigate the meaning of things which the patient brings into the conversation. This is done through the use of open questions and a good ear. Questions that open up and encourage the patient to describe her world for us are, for example, "How was that for you when…?", "What does that mean for you that…?" "How did you experience when…?" "In what way? Can you say more about that?" "How do you mean?" We signal that we are interested in the "voice of the patient", to use Arthur Frank's phrase (Frank 1995).[4]

---

[3] It has been shown that patients are extremely sensitive to giving the "right" answers, and if the professional keeps asking about the objective body it will be the objective body the patient talks about.

[4] Frank writes: "The *postmodern* experience of illness begins when ill people recognize that more is involved in their experiences than the medical story can tell. The loss of a life's map and destination are not medical symptoms, at least until some psychiatric threshold is reached. The scope of modernist medicine—defined in practices ranging from medical school curricula to billing categories—does not include helping patients learn to think differently about their post-illness worlds and construct new relationships to those worlds […] The woman reported by

Questions which close are for example, to ask a fact gathering question, after someone has just given a rich description of their experience, such as "And how often do you need to urinate during the day?" The students role play and tape sessions in the course of learning the method, and it becomes obvious to them that they use questions that "close" down the voice of the patient as an attempt to avoid having to enter the area of the personal, the difficult and the uncomfortable. Clearly, experienced clinicians are beyond this level, but due to the dominance of the objective body and the lack of thematic training, it may feel uncomfortable even for the experienced professional to leave the discussion of the objective body and encourage the patient to speak freely about their experiences.

In conclusion, today's health care institutions must take into account a variety of factors that are not addressed by the medical model. People's health needs today are different from the days when the local GP came to the bedside of the sick person with his little black bag. Whether we like it or not, modern ill health has to do with not only our bodies, but also our psychosocial needs, lifestyle, goals and values. We find ourselves in a time when health is defined as not merely the "absence of disease" yet much of the repertoire for curing ill health rests upon a model where ill health is constituted precisely in terms of material malfunctioning in the somatic body. We need a complementary theory and a new vocabulary that can address the "whole" person in a meaningful way. We also need treatment strategies that can take on the "whole" person, not just the machine-body. It is my hope that the insights of Merleau-Ponty's phenomenology, applied to the area of psychosomatics in this book can provide this much needed new perspective.

Reference

Frank, A. (1995). *The wounded storyteller: Body, illness, and ethics*. Chicago: The University of Chicago Press.

(Footnote 4 continued)
Bourdieu seems to perceive that medicine has taken away her voice: medicine assails her with words she does not want to know and leaves her not knowing what. But this woman does not perceive a need for what would now be called *her own voice*, a personal voice telling what illness has imposed on her and seeking to define for herself a new place in the world. What is distinct in postmodern times is people feeling a need for a voice they can recognize as their own." (pp. 6–7) italics in original.

Index

J. Bullington, *The Expression of the Psychosomatic Body from a Phenomenological Perspective*, SpringerBriefs in Philosophy,
DOI: 10.1007/978-94-007-6498-9, © The Author(s) 2013

The manufacturer's authorised representative in the EU is Springer Nature Customer Service Centre GmbH, Europaplatz 3, 69115 Heidelberg, Germany. If you have any concerns regarding our products, please contact ProductSafety@springernature.com

Printed and bound by CPI Group (UK) Ltd, Croydon, CR0 4YY
01/10/2026
02226351-0012